It Will Change Your Life

A Cochlear Implant Journey

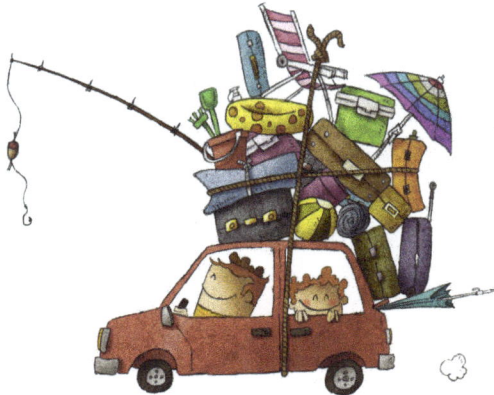

Julieann Wallace

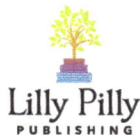

Lilly Pilly
PUBLISHING

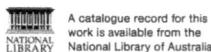

Dedication

To Anne - *thank you for all you do to help people with Meniere's*
To Cochlear Australia - *thank you, my cochlear implant changed my life*
To My Family, Friends and Colleagues - *thank you for being patient with me with my hearing loss before my cochlear implant. Your kindness makes the world a happier place*

Contents

Cochlear Implant Doubt 1

Cochlear Implant Doubt continued 7

Cochlear Implant Assessment 15

My Cochlear Implant Fate 23

The Cochlear Implant Surgeon 31

MRI & CT Scan 37

Psychology Appointment 45

Cochlear Audiologist 57

Balance Rehabilitation 65

Love Letter To My Left Ear 73

Three days before the Cochlear Implant Surgery… 79

One Day Before the Cochlear Implant Surgery… 83

Surgery Day … 87

Anxious 101

Activation Day… 107

It Did Change My Life 109

Learning to Hear 125

My Hearing Addiction 131

Returned Natural Hearing? .137

3 Month Cochlear Implant Mapping 149

It's My Life, My Illness …

    Please Let Me Choose My Treatment 157

One Year Mapping Appointment 169

Two Year Mapping Appointment 175

Cochlear Implant Surgeon Appointment 179

Invitation to Macquarie University 183

Tips for Success With a Cochlear Implant 203

In My Future 208

About the Author 209

Acknowledgements 210

1973. Terror filled me and I covered my ears. The student teacher's lesson was about ears and hearing, and told the class of seven year olds that some people lose their hearing.

Tears filled my eyes and my bottom lip trembled. I never wanted to lose my hearing. I never wanted to go Deaf.

Miss Naomi called me over and put her hand on my shoulder. Seven year old me. 'That won't happen to you. You'll be okay,' she said.

With my lips down-turned, I nodded, believing her.

Except, when I turned 28, I wasn't okay. It had started to happen. I started to lose my hearing.

1995. 'Meniere's disease,' my ENT told me. 'I'm sorry. No cause. No cure. You'll have vertigo episodes, hearing loss in your lower tones, at first, until you will lose all of your hearing. You'll also have ear fullness and tinnitus.'

Be *kind* to yourself ...
intentionally,
extravagantly,
unconditionally.

Monday 21st October, 2019
cochlear implant doubt

The day is overcast, mirroring my mood. Today, I go for a cochlear implant "work-up" for my left ear. I've been considering a cochlear implant for a while, but have bathed in the delusion that somehow, my hearing will come back. But of course, it won't – it's just my eternal hope that floats around me as I journey through the abhorrent, incurable Meniere's disease.

My symptoms started in 1995. Ear fullness, like I had been swimming and still had water stuck in my ear canal. Bouts of unpredictable, violent vertigo. Tinnitus. And then came the hearing loss. Fluctuating at first, until I gradually lost hearing.

It started when I was 28.

'Meniere's is more common in men over 50,' my ENT told me. Online information at the time backed up his statement.

Today, I sit looking out the window at the dark, heavy clouds, painting the state of my heavy heart and dark emotion. I'm 24 years into my Meniere's journey, yet I'm filled with tingles of anxiety travelling over my skin like waves, with one big question bouncing around in my mind. *If I have a cochlear implant, will the disabling **vertigo** of Meniere's disease return?*

That's my fear. When I talk about vertigo, I'm not just talking about being "dizzy". The vertigo of Meniere's disease for me, was the most abhorrent, violent, room spinning.

Totally debilitating.

It was "hold on to the floor or the bed, even though you are already lying on the floor or bed". I had to stare at one spot on the wall for four or five hours until the spinning subsided. And whatever you do, DON'T move your head. It will make the spinning one hundred times worse.

Beyond exhausting. Soul destroying.

And let's not forget the relentless, vicious puking that feels like you're about to turn inside-out, dehydrating the body so much you need to be transported to emergency at the hospital.

If you ever want to know how vertigo of Meniere's feels, sit on an office swivel chair and get someone to spin you around and around and around as fast as they can.

Now, imagine not being able to stop it. Not being able to get off that office chair for hours and hours and hours.

Then imagine, never being able to predict when vertigo will hit – and when it does, you are stuck wherever you are, and you absolutely cannot move, as it will make the spinning impossibly worse. This is the vertigo of Meniere's. Hell.

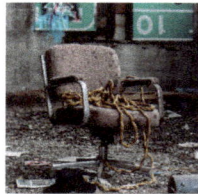

In 2004 I made the choice to destroy the balance cells in

my left ear to stop the debilitating, violent vertigo. The vial of ototoxic gentamicin was now my hope. My ENT injected it into my middle ear through a grommet.

Imagine for one moment, having to make the choice to destroy your balance cells. *Balance*. Yeah – that thing. Something you never even think about. Your body just does it for you.

The day after the gentamicin injection, I woke up with bouncy vision. Every time I took a step, my whole world bounced up and down. I still had balance cells in my right ear, but destroying the balance cells in my left ear made my whole body balance precarious. It's called oscillopsia.

I had to slow down and relearn my new balance, and retaught myself how to walk with a damaged vestibular system. It was my new normal. I learned to use my eyesight as my guide for balance. But compared to the unpredictable vertigo, the destruction to my vestibular system was an answered prayer.

It changed my life. It gave me my life back, with physical limitations. I was no longer spiralling down into the darkness of the Meniere's prison where there was no escape.

But back to my question – *if I have a cochlear implant, will the disabling vertigo return? And if it does, what does it mean for my life after living vertigo free for 15 years?*

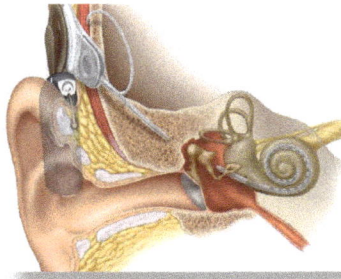

Image St Vincent's Hospital

I'm taking a risk. I know that. The thought of having vertigo again *terrifies* me. My vertigo years were a very, very dark emotional place to be. And I never want to return there.

Once upon a time I lived my life fully – teaching full-time, sport, art, social life, music, holidays, rainforest walks, parties, family events ... it was go, go, go.

I was happy.

Then Meniere's hit and took it all away. Every waking moment was lived in fear of a vertigo attack. Sleep was not even a safe place. I would wake during the night, spinning violently, unable to close my eyes for three or four hours until it stopped.

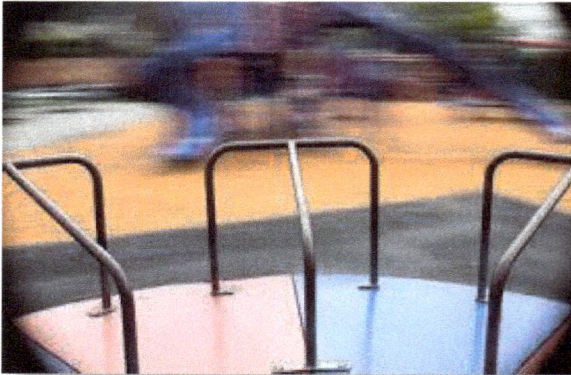

I need answers from my ENT and my Otologist, whom I am yet to see.

Can my Meniere's vertigo return due to the cochlear implant?

I walk out the front door and lock it behind me, my unfriend, Anxiety, joining me for the cochlear implant "work-up" appointment. Anxiety. We have been unfriends for a long time, introduced to each other by my dark, dark shadow, Meniere's disease.

My friends who already have a cochlear implant, tell me it *will change my life* …

I sigh and wonder, which way it will change my life?

Just breathe, I tell myself …

Vertigo is ...
distressing

'Are you spinning, Gram? Is that what's making you sick?'

'Yes ... the room is spinning around me and it won't stop ... it's so fast, Landi, anti-clockwise ... so very fast ...' Gram's lips turned pale and she started to perspire.

I shut my eyes at the sound she made before she vomited hard, once again.

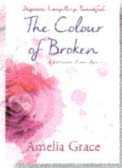

The Colour
of Broken

Amelia Grace

Monday 21st October, 2019
cochlear implant doubt continued …

My self-imposed silence is smothering me. The journey to the cochlear audiologist in the city is forty minutes long. Forty minutes of staring out the window. Looking, but not seeing. Forty minutes of mixed feelings and questions ruminating inside me, alongside anxiety, and the five impossibly loud noises of tinnitus that never leave me.

I can never have inner silence. Peace. *Ever.*

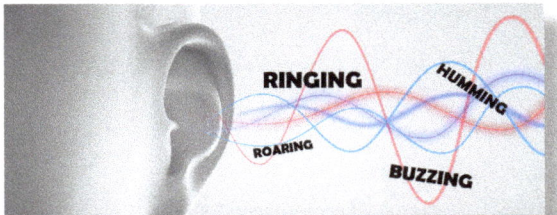

I turn my head towards my husband. My ENT shakes his hand each time we visit him, and he fills him with kind words about sticking by me through my Meniere's journey. 'Most men would have left their wives by now,' the ENT says.

I focus on his facial scars from a recent surgery to remove two skin cancers from the bridge of his nose (a Basal Cell Carcinoma and Squamous Cell Carcinoma). Sixty-eight stitches. 'There goes my modelling career,' he joked with the plastic surgeon. We all laughed. Our fabulous Australian sun loves us too much. At least the cancers are removed now. He'll get on with this life after this slight hiccup like nothing even happened.

It's not as if he has a debilitating condition that stops him from enjoying life, I think.

My stomach drops. I berate myself for not being sympathetic to what he has been through, and guilt hits me like a freight train.

Disappointed with myself, I look back to the road before us, the movement of cars making me nauseous.

I hate Meniere's disease. When will it end? Meniere's for life. Like a prison sentence. Wherever I go, Meniere's goes. My shadow, always present. Lurking.

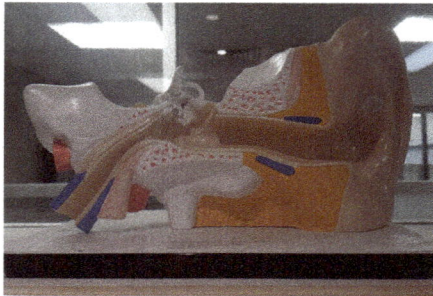

The first thing I see at the hearing centre is a ginormous ear. Yep. I'm at the right place!

An audiologist enters the reception area and calls me to follow him. We go into a soundproof room and he introduces himself, and then asks me, 'Your Meniere's started in which year?'

'My left ear,' I answer.

'Uh – huh. Which … **year** … did it start?' He repeats.

I burst out laughing at my mishearing. *Welcome to my life*.

He doesn't laugh like me. I'm guessing he has heard it all before. I am having my hearing tested for hear loss after all. Mishearing is nothing new to him.

'It started in 1995,' I answer in a serious voice.

He asks more general questions, and at the end of his questioning I say – just for general information, 'I know that research shows no cause and no cure for Meniere's, but I believe my Meniere's is caused by being hit on the side of my head, close to my left ear, by a softball when I was sixteen.'

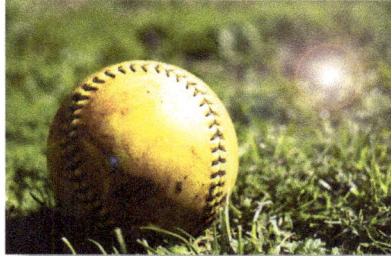

The audiologist leans back in his chair and folds his arms. *Uh-oh…*

He takes a deep breath. 'Meniere's disease is an inflammation of the endolymphatic sac and—'

'I know, in detail, what happens in the inner ear with Meniere's. I have been researching about it for 24 long years and was invited to the Meniere's Symposium in Sydney last year (2018) and have heard about, and seen images of the physiology of what happens during a vertigo attack.' I had cut him off. I feel bad. He assumed I had no idea I knew anything about my disease, as one would. He should have asked first. All of us Menierians search for the exact moment in time that might have *changed our lives*, and research the disease itself. We talk to each other. We know A LOT of stuff about our disease.

He gives me a nod and says no more on the subject.

I add, 'I had a hearing test a couple of years ago and it showed that I have cookie bite hearing loss (cookie bite hearing loss is a special kind of sensorineural hearing loss when a person has problems hearing mid frequency sounds - it's often hereditary). It's genetic on my father's side. That's why I would like to get a cochlear implant, so at least I have some hearing in the future.'

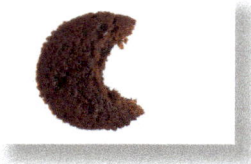

He gives me a nod again. 'Okay. Let's start the hearing test.'

He sets me up with the earphones, beeper, gives me the usual hearing test instructions then sits at his desk of hearing test gear. He gives a sigh.

We begin on my "good" ear first, and I push the button each time I hear a beep, trying to ignore the terribly loud tinnitus in my left ear. Some of the tones I guess, because I don't know if it is the tinnitus sound or the beep, so I just push the button anyway.

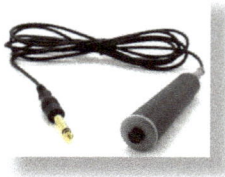

My Meniere's ear is next. I cannot hear the beginning of the beep at any time, but towards the finish of the sound, at times I hear the end of the beep, *I think*, so I press the button. I get excited when I can hear some high tones. I CAN hear! My heart smiles.

The testing continues. By the end, I have sat through the

following hearing tests:

1. Pure tone audiometry, which tests how loud different sounds need to be for you to hear them.

2. Air conduction, which measures whether you can hear different tones played through headphones.

3. Bone conduction, which measures how well your cochlear picks up vibrations.

4. Tympanometry, which isn't a hearing test, but a check of your eardrum.

When the audiologist is finished, I sit in silence and wait on his results, still buzzing from the fact that I could hear some high tones in my Meniere's ear. It is a good day!

He looks up from the audiometric graph and pulls a face. I interpret it as a good result. I **can** hear in my Meniere's ear, when I thought I was profoundly deaf. That's what he is about to tell me …

'You don't have cookie bite hearing loss,' he says. 'Your right ear is fine, except you can't hear the high sounds above our normal hearing range, which people with normal hearing can hear on our tests. Your Meniere's ear is what we call, "dead".'

I am surprised, and happy. *I don't have cookie bite hearing loss? How did the testing show cookie bite hearing loss two years ago at another audiologist appointment, but not now?* I'll take it as a win for my good ear.

Then my heart sinks. Weirdly I feel sorry for my left ear. The audiologist called it "dead".

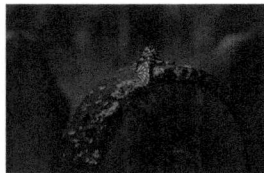

I touch my ear without thinking. Like consoling it. It's like he has hurt its feelings. I blink.

The audiologist continues, 'We do cochlear implants for one-sided hearing loss like yours. You have zero speech discrimination, so a cochlear implant will help you. Are you seeing Jane, the cochlear implant assessor, after this test?'

'No. That's Monday.' I nod. My unfriend, Anxiety, raises its head.

He gives me a smile. 'Right. Let's optimize your Cros hearing aids.'

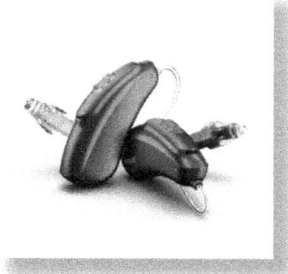

I follow him to another room overlooking the city. He cleans my Phonak Cros hearing aids that I love. I wear two – the left one sends the sound to the right hearing aid, so I can hear sound on my left side.

The audiologist tells me where the best place is for prices to get replacement filters and batteries. Then he places the hearing aids into my ears, puts an analysing device on my shoulders, and connects it all to the computer. He adds my latest hearing results to the program, and just like that, the computer system optimizes my Cros hearing technology. Brilliant.

I walk out of the audiologist's rooms happier than I entered. I don't have the hereditary cookie bite hearing loss that affects only the girls on my dad's side of the family, like my aunty and her three daughters. I'd add a happy skip, but I'd lose my balance and fall over. My shadow, Meniere's, chuckles at me.

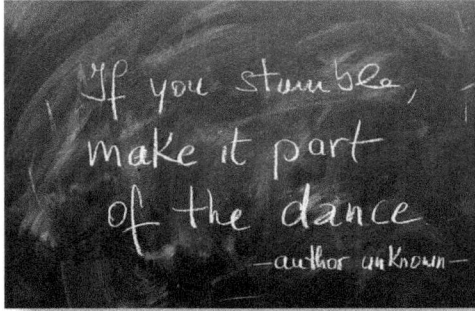

If you stumble,
make it part
of the dance
—author unknown—

Next appointment: *assessment for a cochlear implant …*

Meniere's disease ...
changes everything

'My life is nothing now. I can't work. I can't drive. I can't walk without losing my balance. I can't socialise. I can't hear. I can't eat what I want. My independence has been stripped away. Every moment is lived in fear of a vertigo attack, even while I sleep. I will never hear silence, or peace and quiet again, with the five impossibly loud sounds of tinnitus, incessantly torturing me. Meniere's has taken everything from me ... *everything* ... except family!'

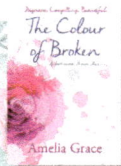

Monday 28th October, 2019
cochlear implant assessment

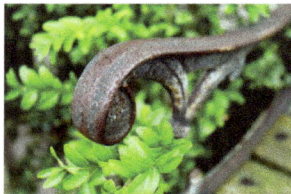

Mum and Dad sit on the garden seat, waiting for me.

I'm having my cochlear implant assessment today. This time I have to drive to the city. Except I can't drive there by myself with 100% confidence. There's too much visual movement and I don't know which direction sound is coming from. Moving my head from side to side makes me nauseous … it's a vestibular and visual nightmare.

I'm tired when we arrive. Being on high alert and concentrating intensely for an hour is exhausting.

But I feel relieved, and sink down into the seat in the reception area at the audiologist. Soon after, Jane greets me with a smile. The universal language that puts you at ease. My unfriends, Anxiety, Tinnitus, Deafness, my shadow – Meniere's, and I follow her to her office. I place my novel, *The Colour of Broken*, onto the desk beside me.

Jane tells me she is the Hearing Implant Manager, and a Senior Lecturer at the School of Health and Rehabilitation Science at the University of Queensland. I am in good hands. She is also the one who decides my fate, whether I am a candidate for a cochlear implant or not.

She reviews my file, my recent hearing test, and questions me about my history with Meniere's disease, taking notes as I talk. Then she opens a power-point on the computer. It explains, page by page, the options for hearing devices for one sided hearing loss, like mine: Cros hearing aids, and the bone conduction implants – BAHA and Bonebridge, commenting that they aren't suitable due to the hearing loss in my "good" ear.

She focuses on the cochlear implant slides: the what, why, how. Afterward, words on the screen bounce out at me like they're in 3D:

"A Cochlear Implant can be the extraordinary alternative that **CHANGES YOUR LIFE!**"

There's those words again. It will *change your life*. I keep reading it. I keep hearing those words from others.

Jane hands me the cochlear implant to hold. *This is really happening.* I heft it. I am surprised by the light weight. She places the outer cochlear components on my head and holds it there so I can feel what it is like.

Small steps, I think. This is a method of easing you into the implant, to help with acceptance. Psychology at work.

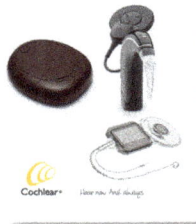

'What do you think? Do you still want a cochlear implant?' she asks.

'Yes,' my unfriend, Anxiety, and I answer. My shadow, Meniere's, glares at me.

'What would a cochlear implant do for you?' she asks.

I frown. What a weird question. *It will help me to hear from my left ear again, obviously*, I think. Is this a trick question? After all, she is the person who will decide whether I am a candidate for a cochlear implant or not.

My shadow, Meniere's, laughs at me.

I take a deep breath. 'It would give other Meniere's people hope of hearing again. It's such a horrid, depressing disease. They need to know that a cochlear implant can help us hear again when they think there is nothing that can be done for hearing … and … I have counselled some people out of suicide. This will give them hope.'

'That's a very heavy burden to carry,' she says.

I frown at her. *Burden?* I have never considered it a burden.

Jane tilts her head to the side a little. 'What … would a cochlear implant do for … *Julieann?*'

And there it is. The question I was avoiding. The question about me. My eyes sting and tears threaten. Stop.

The question is digging deeper than I want it to. I thought I had boxed away all my emotion to do with Meniere's disease. This is meant to be my brave, courageous face. My *Sunday smile*.

The one I wear all the time, so people don't know when I am suffering. I'm a pro at it.

My shadow, Meniere's, chuckles. It's always there, lurking.

I look out the window at the skyscrapers. How do I answer? *What would a cochlear implant do for Julieann – for me?* The obvious answer is that I want to be able to hear in my left ear again.

Am I being selfish? What does Jane want to hear? What are the magic words she wants me to say?

'For me?' I shake my head, not wanting to continue to answer. This question is hurting. Deeply. 'I'm always putting myself last …' I shake my head again. *Do I even deserve to hear again with my Meniere's ear?* I think. *A psychologist would have a field day with that comment!* Tears. Stop. STOP!

I cover my eyes with my fingers to prevent the waterfall of tears running down my face. I can't ugly cry. My mum will notice when I finish the session. I don't want her to know I have been crying … I take a deep breath and sigh, trying to imagine a life of hearing with a cochlear implant … it's so hard to remember what having two hearing ears was like.

I get a brief mind glimpse of the me before Meniere's disease. Before the shadow of darkness took the full, vibrant colour away from my life. I can be re-coloured, right?

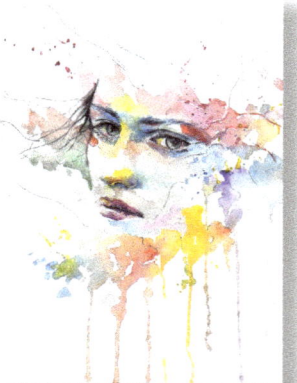

I swallow the lump of emotion rising from my chest. I can't look back at my life. It's too painful. I need to keep looking forward. *Courage. Breathe.*

I look at Jane. Tears trickle.

'A cochlear implant would give me a sense of direction of sound, especially with teaching in the classroom and yard duty. It would be a safety issue at school and my non-school life – my husband has saved me three times from being run over by a car … I would be able to go to social gatherings again. I don't do social events anymore because I can't hear what is being said, and people get tired of me asking them to repeat what they have said. I smile and nod when I shouldn't be, and people frown at me. They choose to talk to someone else because I can't hear them properly. The rejection hurts … *really* hurts. I now choose not to go out with friends and colleagues because I can't hear properly.' The words gush out of me.

'Good,' she says. 'Do you still want a cochlear implant?'

'Yes,' I whisper.

'Let's do some hearing tests,' she says. I'm baffled. I did a thorough hearing test less than a week ago.

Wearing my Phonak Cros hearing aids, I sit between two large speakers, one near my left ear, the other one near my right. Jane tells me to keep looking forward and not to move my head.

Sentences flow out of the speakers that I have to repeat. First with no background noise, and then with background noise on my left, and then on my right.

Even with my Cros aids on, I don't have any speech discrimination when background noise is played on my good ear side. I do however get one sentence right – 'Are you baking chocolate cake for the visitors tonight?' I feel pleased with myself. My chocoholicism is shining through.

'You're very good at keeping your head still,' she says.

'I've had lots of practice.' The memory of spinning violently with vertigo comes crashing forward. How many days have I walked around and not moved my head to stop the nausea, or trying to put off an impending vertigo attack? How many hundreds/thousands of hours have I keep my head perfectly still while spinning and staring at a spot on the wall for 3 or 4 or more hours while spinning?

'You're very good at focussing on the words with the background noise playing,' she says.

'I've had lots of practice,' I answer, thinking, *this is every moment of my awake life.*

'If you are given a cochlear implant, you have to work at learning to listen with it. It's not a magical device that's turned on and suddenly you can hear normally. You must have people around you who will support you.'

She looks at the empty chair in the room. I take the cue and babble on about my husband having to go back to work today after facial surgery, and that my mum and dad are waiting outside for me.

'Thanks, Julieann. I'll write up a report about my recommendation for you and send it to your ENT. He will tell you if you are a candidate for the cochlear implant.'

Relief washes over me. I am done. No more tests or questions that are too uncomfortable for me to answer.

I gesture toward my novel.

'I'd like to give this book to everyone here. It has a main character with Meniere's disease. I wrote it to raise awareness and to help raise money to find a cure. I've donated around $3,200 to Meniere's research so far. Amelia Grace is my pen name.'

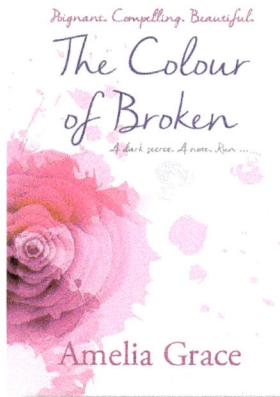

Jane smiles and I sign it – "*The spark of hope can never be extinguished*".

'I'll leave it in a place for all patients to be able to read, but I'm going to be the first person to read it!' She looks at me, her eyes twinkling.

I walk out of the consultation – me and my shadow, Meniere's. My unfriend, Anxiety, is dawdling behind. Tinnitus is skipping and Deafness has no idea what is going on. Jane hands me a yellow folder.

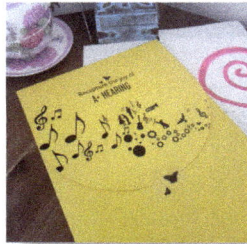

The moment my mum and dad see me they smile ... the universal language that puts you at ease, and I hope they can't see the streaks of tears that I cried.

Next appointment: *back to my ENT to learn my fate.*

Vertigo is ...
a betrayal of the body

Gram vomited. Violently. I handed her a tissue and she wiped her mouth and dropped it into the container.

'I hate this ... I hate this damn disease—' Gram vomited once again.

I sat on the floor, holding her hand. 'How long have you been like this, Gram?'

'Five and a half hours of the room spinning around me and vomiting, of staring at the same place on the damn wall to try to stop the bloody vertigo.' She took short breaths, breathing them out forcefully between pursed lips. Her wide eyes were filled with fear. 'The most ridiculous thing is ... I know the room is not spinning, yet, everything in my damn body and mind tells me it is. It's such a lie ... *a lie!*'

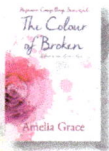

The Colour
of Broken

Amelia Grace

Thursday October 31st, 2019
my cochlear implant fate

I'm filled with so much doubt. I am *choosing* to get a cochlear implant. Am I allowed to choose? Or should I just accept my fate that I will remain without hearing for the length of my days, auditory colour disappearing from my life.

I didn't *choose* to have Meniere's disease. I didn't *choose* vertigo. I didn't *choose* deafness. I didn't *choose* tinnitus. Just like other people who didn't choose their incurable diseases or illnesses.

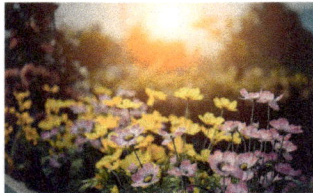

A cochlear implant feels like a second chance. A second chance at hearing, of taking back something Meniere's disease has taken from me. In my mind's eye, I am facing the beast of Meniere's, my sword drawn.

I want to be violent with Meniere's. So violent. I hate it. I hate what it has done to me. What it has taken from me. I hate what it does to its victims. I want to slay it with an intensity that will obliterate it for eternity, with such force that it withdraws from bodily habitation of every person who suffers from it.

Cure, come soon.

Please.

I arrive in the city. I look up briefly from the footpath that I walk on. A rarity. My normal walk is focussed on the ground in front of me, ensuring each step will keep my balance. I see an old windmill on top of the terrace. Unkempt grey, striking against the beautiful lilacs of the Jacaranda tree. It was built by the convicts in the late 1820s and is the oldest windmill in existence in Australia. Due to its windless location, the windmill morphed into a symbol of "dread and torture" as penal Commandant Patrick Logan used convicts to work a treadmill he had constructed to keep the arms turning in lieu of wind.

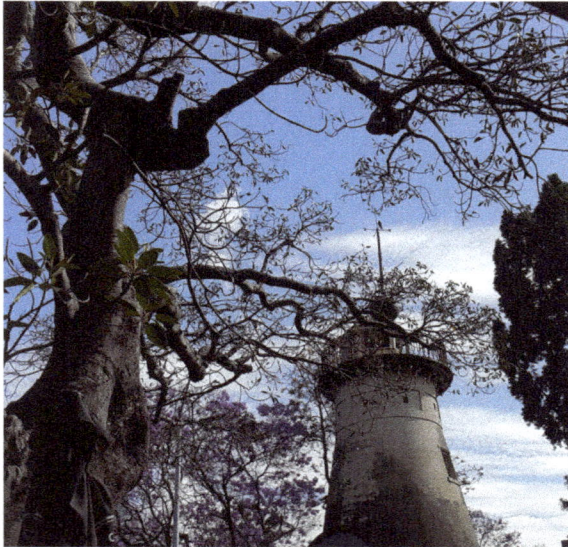

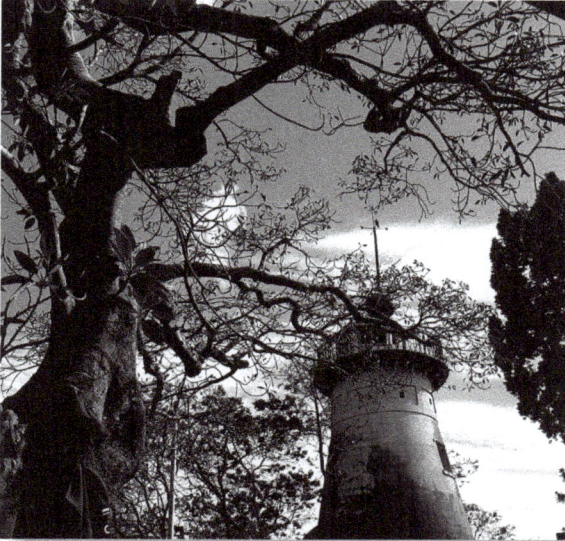

Dread and torture. Fitting. A perfect symbol for Meniere's disease.

A weather-vane decorates the uppermost part of the windmill. And there sits a crow, blacker than night. It squawks. *Welcome*, I hear. *Today, you will learn of your fate.*

I inhale deeply. My eyesight returns to the uneven, battered, cracked path in front of me. Falling is never a good thing. Once you have your balance cells destroyed, when you fall, you have no idea where to place your hands to protect yourself.

The first time I fell was Christmas, 2018. My family and I were on holidays in Tasmania, walking the Dove Lake trek at Cradle Mountain. 5.7 km. 3 hours.

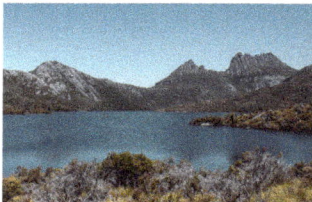
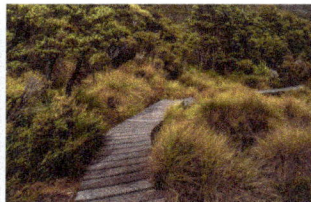

After the walk we entered the cafeteria for a drink. Without warning, tears filled my eyes. In public.

My husband turned to me and the look on his face said it all. His eyes widened. 'What's wrong?'

'I fell,' I said. I wanted to sob. Loudly. Aftershock from the fall. I caught the sob in my throat. 'I fell and I couldn't stop it.'

His eyes filled with tears, but they didn't leak down his cheek like mine. I always hate seeing his eyes that way. He was following me as we walked, to catch me if I fell. He always does that for me. My protector. And when it happened, I tripped on a step, there was no way he could stop it. I remember the panic in his voice as he leaned over me, asking if I was okay, looking over me, again and again. 'Did you hurt yourself?' he had asked.

All I could say was, 'My phone is under the bush, over there.' I had no idea how I saw it slide under the bush. When I fall I have no idea where to put my hands to stop me, or protect me – inside my head as I'm falling, I see myself as a body but no arms or legs. That's what destroying my balance cells did to me. I just have to wait for impact and suffer the consequences.

'I don't care about your phone. Are you okay?' he said.

'Yes,' I said. *It was a lie.* I was hurt. But I wanted to get up to save face. There were many people on the walking track.

I HATE YOU MENIERE'S!

My husband pulled me up off the ground. My daughter picked up my phone. She was too quiet. How many times had she witnessed Meniere's bring me to my knees with vertigo, deafness, depression? And now falling.

I blew out a long breath between my lips. Then set a rock in my sights to sit on for a moment to assess my injuries, then walked there, my husband holding onto my arm to support me. I wanted to yell at him, "LET GO OF ME! I'M NOT AN

INVALID!" But I didn't. He was trying to help.

I sat on the rock, looked over the lake and focussed on where I hurt – my wrist, my arm, my ankle and my back. *Hold yourself together*, I thought, *people fall all the time. Put on your "I'm okay mask"*.

'Are you alright, Ma?' my daughter asked.

Hold yourself together. The emotion of "I want to fall to pieces" rolled through me. *Hold it together. Breathe.*

'It could be worse,' I said, 'I could have broken something.' I was hoping that I didn't break anything. My wrist, arm and ankle were throbbing. Not to mention my back spasms. 'Thanks for picking up my phone,' I added.

She nodded, looking at me with concern in her eyes.

'I'm sorry for falling,' I say to her. I don't want her to be embarrassed by me.

I HATE YOU MENIERE'S!

And of course, she is not. She never is. She's always one of the first to help. It is my own self-judgement that betrays me.

I stand. In pain. But I can walk to finish the last hour of the track.

My daughter is in front of me, glancing back at me every once and a while, and my husband behind me. I'm glad. He can't see me wriggling my fingers to check my wrist, and feeling where my right arm hurts, nor the wince on my face when my ankle hurts more than I want it to, or my back spasms. All I can think of is when my son would roll his ankle at elite triathlon training, and his coach would tell him to walk normally on it. So that is what I do, despite the pain.

Back at the cafeteria …

'I could have died if I fell in a different part of the walk,' I say. It was true. Parts of the track were on a boardwalk above the ground that fell steeply, scattered with rocks and trees below, no rails to stop a tumble.

'I know,' my husband whispered. I watch his watery eyes and see him swallow harder than usual. 'What do you want to drink? Do you want an ice-cream?' He was using the distraction method. He knows me well.

Claire and I find a table away from most of the people. My wrist and arm throb. My back was spasming and my ankle twinging. Swelling was setting in. I ate my ice-cream, flicking tears from my eyes when they dropped. *At least I don't have vertigo*, I thought. It *was* a good day, after all. Any day without vertigo is a good day. *Suck it up*, I tell myself, *it could be worse.*

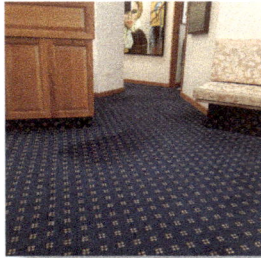

My husband and I enter the ENT's reception area. I laugh, then shake my head in disbelief at the choice of carpet. The pattern on it makes me nauseous – thanks to my shadow, Meniere's.

My ENT calls me in. 'Good news,' he says. 'You are a candidate for a cochlear implant. I have signed you off on it if you wish to proceed.'

I swallow. There it is again. I get to *choose*.

I nod. But not with confidence. More like a "roll with the wave" type of nod. I'm following a path but not certain of that is where I am meant to be. How will it change my life?

He refers me to a cochlear implant surgeon, and then as I leave, I thank him for his support throughout my Meniere's journey.

'You don't know how difficult it has been for me, when there was nothing I could do to help you,' he says.

'But I am one of your success stories,' I remind him. 'I wouldn't be standing here today if it wasn't for your help.'

He kisses my cheek. 'Keep in touch. I want to know how you go.' He gives me a smile. Why does this feel like a goodbye?

I walk out of his office and numbness sets in. I'm a cochlear implant candidate.

This just became very real.

Next appointment: *the cochlear implant surgeon.*

Meniere's disease is ...

personality changing

'Would you like a cup of tea, Gram?'

Grandmother Fleur turned her body towards me like her head was fused in place. It was an odd, robotic type of movement. 'That would be wonderful, Landi. I think I will sit down in the office for a bit.' Her voice was flat, not the cheerful, uplifting voice we were used to.

I watched her walk away. There was no bounce in her step. It was almost a smooth shuffle, and looked like an attempt to walk without making any body movement of any kind.

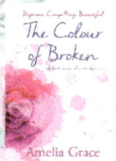

Tuesday November 5th, 2019
the cochlear implant surgeon

Life with an invisible illness is an interesting voyage. People cannot see what you are going through, what you suffer - physically, emotionally, psychologically, socially – your invisible scars – so it's hard for others to empathize.

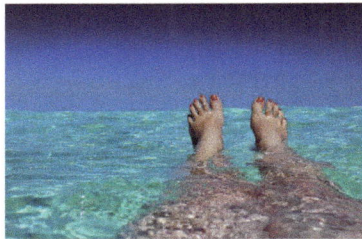

People would often say to me, 'Your life has been so easy. Everything just falls into place. Good things always happen to you. You're always smiling.' It used to frustrate me. They had no idea what I was going through. They had no idea how hard I worked to be where I was in my career, my family, my three children. Nothing ever "fell into place". Every moment of it was earned.

During the hardest time of my Meniere's disease, I was in very deep and dark depression that I couldn't climb out of. Yet, I kept smiling. It was easier that way. I would patch up the cracks in my mask before I put it on, and then met with others. *If I could meet others … if my shadow, Meniere's, hadn't imprisoned me for three, four or five hours of violent, debilitating spinning that would land me in hospital at times.*

In hindsight, I'm glad my illness is invisible. It makes it easier to pretend that I am okay. I don't have people avoiding me like I have a contagious condition. I don't have people looking at me with well-meaning concern, or that "pity" look. I hate the pity look. I don't want to have people devaluing the severity of my symptoms, like:

'It's okay, dear, we all get dizzy sometimes.'

'Oh, I have tinnitus too. It's so common. When it's really quiet, I can hear a little "sssssssssss". You'll be fine!'

'My friend had Meniere's disease – he got a bit faint sometimes. He went to the doctor and is cured.'

Meniere's disease. No cause. No cure. *Yet.*

Good things are coming. I know it. I follow the research.

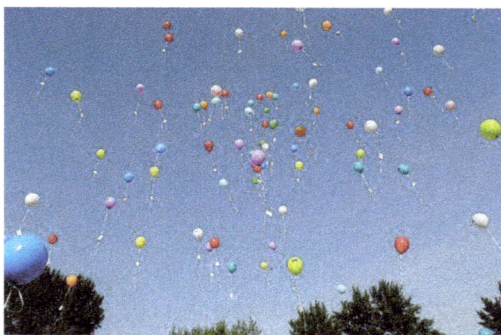

My cochlear surgeon is younger than me, as my ENT had said.

I follow the surgeon into his office, my shadow, Meniere's, behind me, then my husband, and my unfriends, Anxiety and Deafness, far behind. The more I know about the cochlear implant the less anxious I feel. And I am so thankful to many people with cochlear implants who have reached out to me. The world is a wonderful place.

The surgeon tells me that my ENT believes my Meniere's disease has "burnt out".

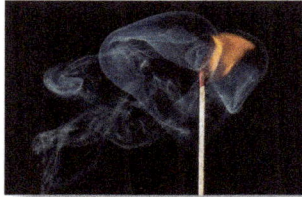

"Burnt out". There's those two words that float around in Meniere's groups.

According to menieres-disease.co.uk, "the term 'burn out' is frequently used to describe Meniere's as though it is the end of the line, that it has finished. However, it really means that the vertigo attacks have disappeared as the vestibular function has now been destroyed. The disease continues to progress as hearing is completely lost, tinnitus and fullness will continue, even after burn out."

'Hmmm … I'm not so sure that it has burned out. I still get little mini spins at times,' I say. And it's definitely not BPPV.

I am questioned about the history of my Meniere's, then the surgeon asks me to sit on a stool so he can look inside my ears.

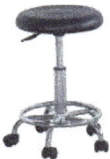

'Spin to your left,' he says.

'Spin?' I say with a smirk, referring to the spinning of vertigo, then swivel the chair to the left, slowly.

'Turn to your left,' he says, smiling. *Ah*

– he has a sense of humour. Good. He uses the auriscope to look inside my ear canal.

'*Turn* … to your right,' he says with a smile in his voice. I swivel the chair to the right, slowly, and he checks inside my ear canal.

The remainder of the appointment flows with quick succession:

Surgery date: 19 December. Overnight stay.

$25, 000 - the cochlear implant cost is covered by the health fund. Any questions?

I take a deep breath. 'Will my vertigo return?'

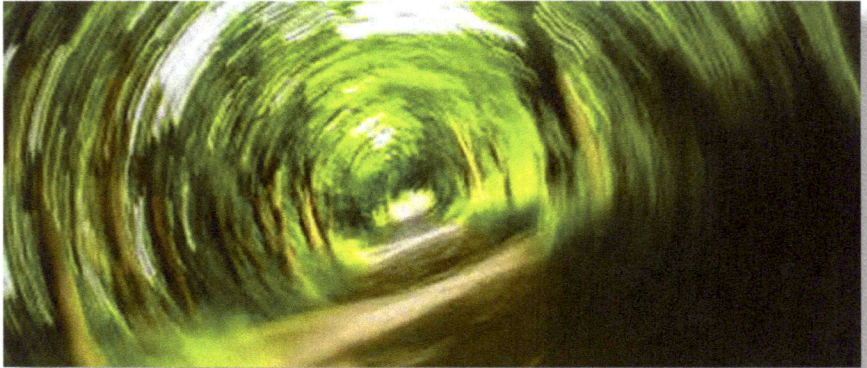

He considers my question, then says, 'I don't expect it to, but there are no guarantees. For Meniere's patients who still have some balance cells left, I usually wash out the inner ear with gentamicin while I am in there as an insurance that they will not have vertigo anymore, but since you have been so good for quite a while without vertigo, I won't do that, in case it upsets anything.'

I nod, feeling a little numb. There is still no certainty that my vertigo will not return. *How can it be burnt out if the vertigo returns?*

My shadow, Meniere's, crosses its arms and grins.

Before I leave, the surgeon gives me a form for an MRI and CT Scan, and tells me I need balance rehabilitation before I have surgery, and to continue afterward.

I raise my eyebrows and nod. I have never had balance rehabilitation; I just relearned my balance to walk by myself after the gentamicin was injected into my middle ear in 2004.

I leave the surgeon's office.

My unfriend, Anxiety, is waiting.

Next appointment: *MRI and CT scan*

Meniere's disease is ... difficult

'Grampapa, hi.'

'Hi back, Yolande.' He looked around the flower store. 'It looks busy this morning,' he said.

'It hasn't stopped since I opened the doors. How's Gram?'

Gramps closed his eyes for more than a moment. 'Still nauseous ... scared.'

'Scared?'

'Of another vertigo attack.' Gramps brushed his hand over his face. When he moved his hand away, he shook his head. His eyes were wet.

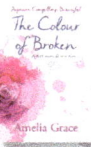

The Colour of Broken

Amelia Grace

Thursday November 7, 2019
MRI & CT scan

My beautiful daughter, Claire, is driving her beloved Mini. I'm sitting beside her, groovy sunglasses on. My shadow, Meniere's, is bouncing up and down on the seat behind me like a child high on sugar. My unfriend, Anxiety, sits beside him, shaking its head at Meniere's. I smirk at Anxiety. Deafness sits quietly.

We are on the way to my MRI and CT Scan. Claire volunteered to drive me. She has always loved Minis. Her love affair began a long time ago, way before she had her Year 12 Formal in 2015, when we hired a Mini convertible to drive her and a friend to the formal venue.

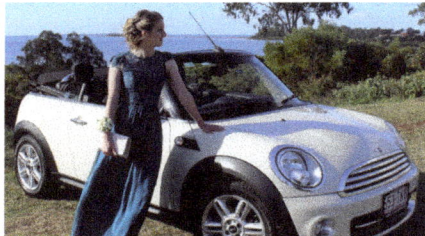

Claire has a heart of gold. I often feel guilty that I couldn't give her and her two brothers a childhood of excitement like I had always dreamed of because of my Meniere's disease. They missed out on Wiggles concerts, other concerts, rides, play dates, adventures etc. Yet, she has grown into a remarkable young woman, and her two brothers are remarkable young men.

We turn the corner into the X-Ray building carpark.

'Do you think they'll find the Meniere's Monster inside my ear on the scans?' I ask.

My shadow, Meniere's, stops bouncing up and down and listens.

'Yes,' replies Claire, 'eating cookies!'

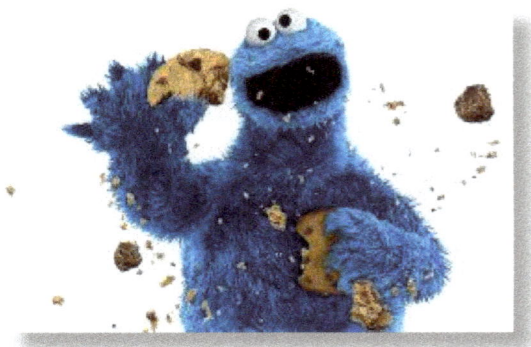

I laugh. That's how we always deal with the cruel Meniere's disease. With humour. 'I don't have cookie bite hearing loss anymore, remember, so it can't be eating the cookies!'

My shadow, Meniere's, pulls a sad face.

Claire smiles at me. She parks her Mini and a mature-aged man smiles at us. *He must love Minis, too*, I think.

Claire is armed with a book to read as she waits for the 40 minute MRI followed by the CT scan.

Today, I have a wandering headache and for once I am glad. I visualise the MRI and CT Scan zapping it to make it go away. I am happy for this next step before the cochlear implant, because if there is anything else nasty going on inside my head, it will show up on the tests.

I wait next to Claire. The waiting room is filled with 60, 70, 80 and 90-year-olds. I feel young for once.

'If you hear my name called, and I don't, can you tell me, please,' I say to Claire. She has always been a source of extra ears for me. So thankful.

My name is called, and surprisingly, I hear it. But then, I have no idea where the voice is coming from. This is the problem with one sided hearing loss, you lose all sense of direction of hearing. It is most frustrating.

I stand and look around the room to match a person and a voice. After scanning the entire area, I see a woman in a QLD X-ray uniform, smiling and waiting at double glass doors. I follow her through the doors and my shadow, Meniere's, follows me with a sassy walk. My unfriend, Anxiety, gives him a poke, and Deafness is oblivious.

After the wardrobe change into the stunning medical attire, I sit and wait. The most interesting thing in the room is the fish tank next to me.

A person appears in front of me, giving me a fright. She approached me from my left side and I didn't hear her. I follow her, with my entourage, into the room with the MRI machine.

Amazing technology.

Before I came to the appointment, I wondered what the difference was between an MRI and a CT Scan, so I Googled it, and found this interesting image that explains it well.

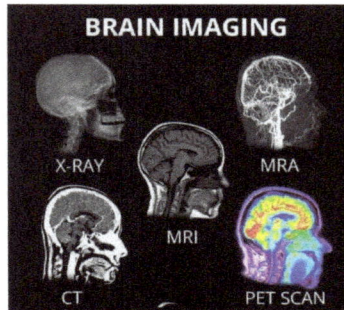

I lie down, put yellow ear plugs into my ears, and then have earmuffs placed over my ears, "to protect my hearing" they say. I chuckle, thinking, *I don't need it for my left ear.*

'You can keep your eyes open or closed, but just don't move your head,' I'm told.

Too easy, I think, *I've had lots of practise at not moving my head. Haven't I, Vertigo?* My shadow, Meniere's, nods.

I'm transported inside the MRI machine.

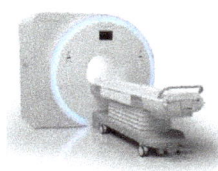

There is nothing but whiteness, except for a picture of fish in their blue water of paradise above me. *Well played*, I think, *giving people something to look at while having an inside picture taken.*

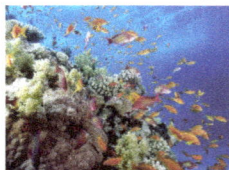

I close my eyes and wait. My tinnitus is loud. The machine is loud, even through the protection of the ear plugs and earmuffs. But my tinnitus is much louder than the MRI machine. Tinnitus is such a show-off, always being the loudest, even at rock concerts.

I frown. Can I hear music? A little. I open my eyes to try and work out the song. "Welcome to the hotel California". *Apt lyrics,* I think, especially the end of the song … *You can check out any time you like, But you can never leave!* Meniere's – you can never leave. I smile with my eyes. Music mirroring life. I look to the fish and decide to count them. 276.

I try to concentrate on hearing more of the music, but I can't. My tinnitus is just too loud.

My shadow, Meniere's, is doing the victory dance.

My Meniere's ear is throbbing, I notice. But not with pain. Is it the earmuff pressure? I shrug in my mind, then imagine the Meniere's monster taking on different poses for selfies with the MRI.

My shadow, Meniere's, takes a bow.

After 20 minutes, the MRI is finished and I go for my CT scan, which is much quicker.

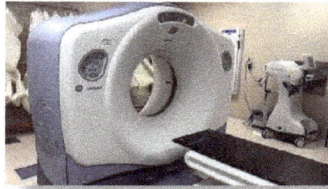

When I leave the building with Claire she asks, 'Did you see any cats in the CT scan?' I give her a big smile.

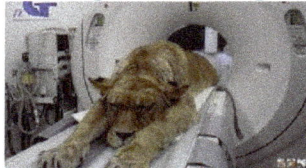

We climb into Claire's Mini and start it up. My shadow, Meniere's, is gazing out the window and my unfriend, Anxiety, has shrunk to the size of a peanut. Tinnitus is playing it's own loud sound and Deafness is looking out the window.

Next destination, shopping. Claire is an artist and has her final art exhibition for university next week. She has a quest – to find something special to wear.

We stop for a hot drink. I choose a lavender latte. A celebration of my next step towards a cochlear implant completed.

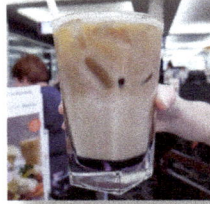

Next appointment: *the psychologist*

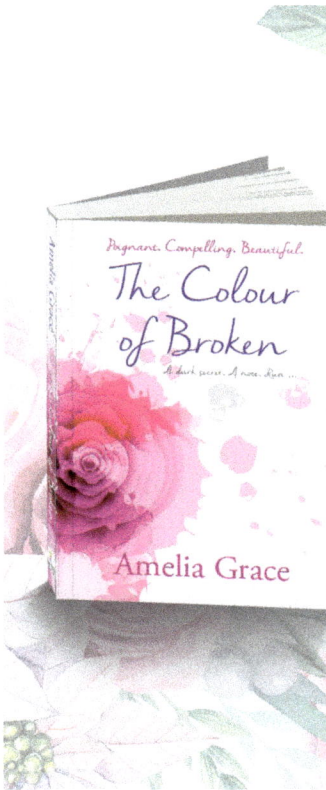

Poignant. Compelling. Beautiful.

The Colour of Broken

A dark secret. A rose. Hope ...

Amelia Grace

'I see people in ... colours ...' I said.

'How long have you seen people this way?'

'Since I was seven.'

'What colour are you?' asked Dr Jones.

I took a deep breath and twisted my fingers together. My stomach tightened. I cleared my throat. 'The colour of broken ...'

Dr Jones was silent.

I stopped breathing when anxiety rose inside me like a wall of lava, about to incinerate me.

'And what colour would that be?' she finally asked.

'It's a crackled dark gray, with other colours that seep out ... sometimes.'

'What colours would they be?'

'Drips of red for anger ... specks of black—' *for self-hate,* '—for my secret, blushes of pink for my love for Mia and my family, and explosions of turquoise that screams at me to love myself ...'

Vertigo is ...

unbearable

'I can't do this anymore ...
Please help me ...
Please help me ...
I can't do this anymore ...'

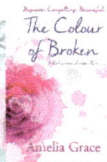

Monday 18th November, 2019
psychology appointment

I see the psychologist today.
How does that make me feel?

When I first started the cochlear implant process, I was informed about the CI "Team":

* ENT. *done*
* Audiologist. *done*
* Surgeon. *done*
* Psychologist …
* Cochlear Audiologist …
* Balance Rehabilitation – *an added one just for me* – only because I have had all my balance cells destroyed in my left ear.

I'm working my way through the list.

I arrive for my appointment ten minutes early, laughing on the inside. I got lost on the way. How can I still be early? My weird sense of humour is getting the better of me. In my best-selling novel, *The Colour of Broken*, the main character, Andi, visits her psychologist regularly. To write the novel, I did a considerable amount of research to ensure the psychologist in my novel was asking the right questions. I already know what to expect.

I open the door and scan the waiting room. I have never seen so many artworks on medical walls. I'm in an artist's paradise.

I'm asked to fill out some paperwork, and I promptly complete it.

Then I have a moment of downtime and the realisation hits me – the psychologist holds a power over me. He is a cog in the wheel of the Cochlear Implant Team who can allow or deny my access to the hearing technology. He will make a judgement call by the end of the session.

I sigh and remind myself, "it's part of the journey", and the Cochlear Implant Team want to ensure my mental wellness.

I open my iPad and work on a Meniere's illustration I have been creating. It's full of symbolism. The buzzing bee for tinnitus. The vertigo flowers for vertigo, and the butterfly for loss of hearing, as most butterflies are deaf. The blue sky is a good coping day.

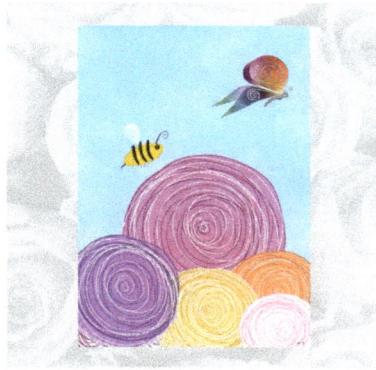

I change the backgrounds to add an oncoming vertigo attack.

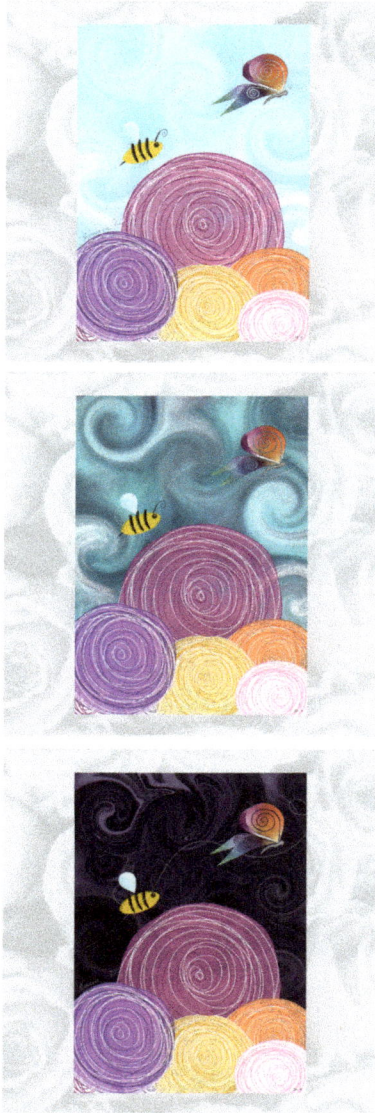

I close my iPad, then soak in time like I have slowed it down. It feels like I have been here before, all because of my novel. It

feels like a book paralleling real life.
Excerpt from *The Colour of Broken*

Poignant. Compelling. Beautiful.
The Colour of Broken
A dark secret. A new life...
Amelia Grace

I sat in the chair outside the psychologist's office. I'm sure it had a permanent imprint of my butt on it. My mother's hand was around my upper arm like a vice so I couldn't run. She knew me well. Thank God. I didn't want to be here, but I did. I needed to be here. Darkness had reached up to pull me under, yet again.

(me in real life)

I sat in the chair outside the psychologist's office. The seat was really comfy and I wiggled down into it. I was here by myself. I didn't want to be here, but I had to. I needed to be here to prove that I was a suitable candidate for a cochlear implant.

(from "The Colour of Broken")

'Yolande.' Dr Jones's voice was comforting, like a warm childhood blankie and a mug of hot chocolate by the fireplace. My mother's grip loosened on my arm and I stood, eyes focussed on the floor. I took slow steps into the office. The familiar office. I'd been here so often I was wondering when she'd ask me to pay rent.

Dr Jones put a light hand on my shoulder and led me to the couch. Usually she asked me whether I wanted to sit on the chair or lie on the couch. Today there was no such question. She knew me well. For a moment I wondered if psychologists ever saw a psychiatrist or psychologist themselves? Who did they go to when they had a problem?

(me in real life)

'Julieann.' The psychologist's voice was hard to hear, like listening to a voice through a wall. I stood, dropping my jacket and pen onto the floor, as per usual, picked them up, then took slow steps into the office. The unfamiliar office. It was smaller than I had imagined. The psychologist gestured to the black sofa with red and blue cushions, and told me to take a seat. I briefly wondered if he has already analysed my conscious choice about where to sit on the sofa. My shadow, Meniere's, sits beside me, and looks the psychologist up and down. I gaze up at the artwork on the wall behind him and comment on the castle sitting on top of a mountain. It has dark undertones. I like it.

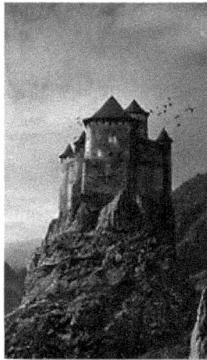

(from "The Colour of Broken")

'*What brings you here today, Andi?*' Dr Jones asked, sitting beside me, so we weren't facing each other.

'*The darkness within,*' I said, and sipped on some more tea. '*And fear.'*

'Ah … good old Darius Darkness. Your friend. What is he trying to tell you?'

'I deserve everything that happened. I almost believed him. But Darius is such a liar. He's relentless at times.'

'Well done, Andi. So, I'm assuming fear has jumped on board to weigh you down?'

'Yes.' I sipped on my tea. It warmed my throat and my stomach. I welcomed its warmth.

'Fear of?'

'Gram wants me to go to a garden party with a stranger to protect her bicycle. She told me not to wear my steel-capped boots.'

'How does that make you feel?'

(me in real life)

'What brings you here today, Julieann?' The psychologist asks, sitting opposite me, so we were facing each other.

I stop a smirk from appearing on my face, and think, he knows exactly why I am here. 'The cochlear audiologist, the surgeon and the ENT,' I rattle off, feeling like I am telling an accumulative story. I wished I had some tea to sip.

'Ah, yes,' he says. 'Getting a cochlear implant will change your life. It's my role is to make sure that you will be able to cope with the change.'

I nod.

'How does getting a cochlear implant make you feel?' he asks.

'I … it …' I look to the floor trying to find the right words. 'I think it will make me feel like I have been released from the Meniere's prison. Having an incurable disease – for anyone – is like feeling captive. You can't leave. You're never free.'

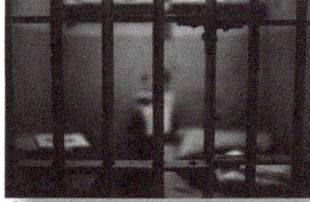

He nods his head as he writes furiously on his paper with a hot pink pen.

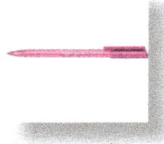

'I think … it feels like … I might get a bit of the old me back, the me before I had Meniere's disease,' I add.

He nods and writes.

'How does that make you feel?'

Silence. I don't want to think back to before I was 30. I finally answer, 'Scared.'

'Why is that?'

'It will push me out of my comfort zone. Sometimes I think people can get comfortable sitting within their disease, and use it as a type of crutch.'

He nods and writes.

His next questions are about my cochlear implant expectations, support people, then he encourages me to describe my life after I get a cochlear implant.

He talks about the importance of resilience, and wants to know what my strategies will be to help me get through it, if somehow, the cochlear implantation isn't what I think it will be.

His next question stops me in my tracks. 'Tell me about your life before Meniere's, and then during Meniere's. I want to know what strategies you used to cope when you had active Meniere's.

My voice trembles as I recount my life before Meniere's. I never like reminiscing about what is was like being free of the beast. And I hate reminiscing about the very dark time in my life with active Meniere's.

Tears. Stop. I manage to keep my tears strategically balancing on my eyelids.

I take a deep breath then I tell him I would wake up each day and look for the positives. Even the very small positives, like the colour of flowers and nature. Petting my dog. I tell him I write, and it helps me. It's the only time I don't hear the loud tinnitus. I tell him I have a published novel with a main character with Meniere's to raise awareness and help others that has sold around 2000 copies. I tell him that I volunteer as a research subject when the Mind and Brain Centre at the University of Queensland puts a call out for Meniere's people. I tell him that I love art, and recently exhibited a series of 4 artworks for Meniere's awareness, called 'Captive'.

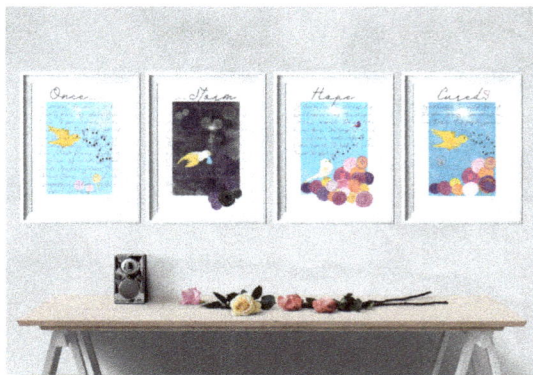

The psychologist is writing at a phenomenal rate. I wonder if he has his own type of shorthand. Then I wonder if he can always read his words afterward.

For a split second in time I want to say, 'You're using a pink pen. How does that make you feel?' But I don't. Instead, I search my mind for the meaning of pink – "the colour pink is the colour of universal love of oneself and of others". He is in the right profession.

He stops writing and looks at me. 'You would make an interesting research subject with something psychologists have recently termed "post-traumatic growth", where you can use all the negativity of what has happened to you and use in a positive way.'

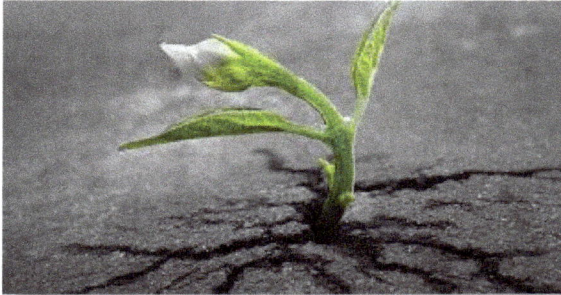

I half smile. I would have preferred *not* having an incurable disease in the first place. I want to tell him that I discovered "post-traumatic growth" all by myself, and didn't need a psychologist to give me the strategy or the label. I want to say that realistically, humans have been "post-traumatic growth-ing" since the beginning of trauma. It's one way we bring light back into our dark world.

The psychologist leans back in his chair. 'My job now is to write a report and send it to the Cochlear Implant Team. I will recommend that you are a suitable candidate for a cochlear implant, and that you have strategies that will help you cope with the change that is coming.'

I smile. 'Thank you,' I say, then pluck up the courage to comment on a piece of artwork the room. I know it is part of the ink blot test.

He smiles back. 'It's from Rorschach's Ink Blot test.' Then he takes me to the reception area and proudly shows me the Rorschach's Ink Blot Test Collection – on a background of typed text, mounted and framed.

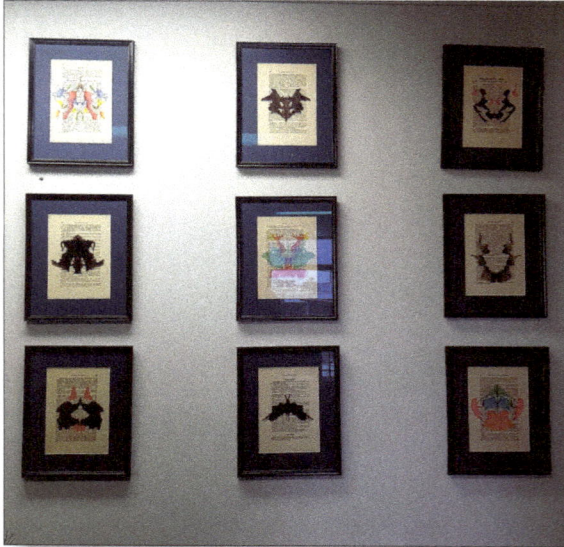

If Meniere's disease was one of those ink blots, it would definitely be:

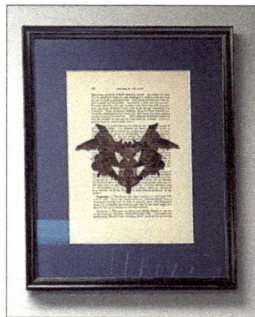

I leave the psychology appointment with a bounce in my

step. The cochlear implant is getting closer to becoming a reality.

I have also finalised the design of my Meniere's artwork in my mind that I was working on before the meeting, and go home and finish it.

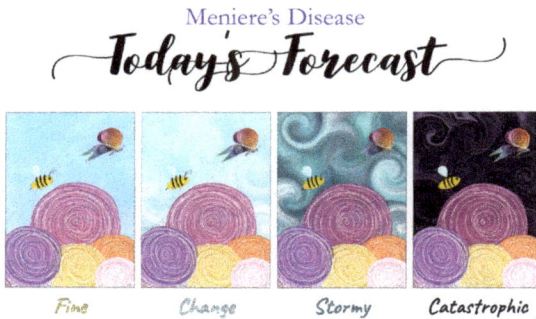

Next appointment: *final expectations with the cochlear audiologist.*

Meniere's disease is ...
a weather predictor

I turned my head toward Gram. Her walk was unsteady, like she had had a few too many drinks. *Did she?* I watched as she turned, keeping her entire body stiff as she did so.

She stopped beside me and put her hand on my back. 'The rain is coming, Landi. Put the umbrellas out.'

'But it's sunny outside!'

'Trust me. It's going ... to rain. My brain fog is back, and my ear feels full, the tinnitus is roaring, and moving my head is like doing it in slow motion, plus it makes me feel nauseous. The rain ... is coming.'

'Oh, Gram. I had no idea the weather affected you like that.'

'Just another wonderful part of this disease—the unique meteorologist ability it grants ...'

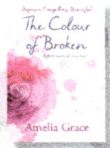

The Colour of Broken

Amelia Grace

Wednesday 20th November, 2019
cochlear audiologist

I'm feeling super nervous today. My unfriend, Anxiety, has grown bigger than me, and my shadow, Meniere's, is using it as a punching bag while Tinnitus whistles. Deafness observes closely. I have an appointment with the cochlear implant audiologist to discuss "final expectations". This is my do or die day. My "yes, let's do it day", or, "I've changed my mind, I've decided not to go ahead with the procedure day".

Do I really want to take the step into the bionic hearing world? *Am I brave enough?* I just want to sit and cry.

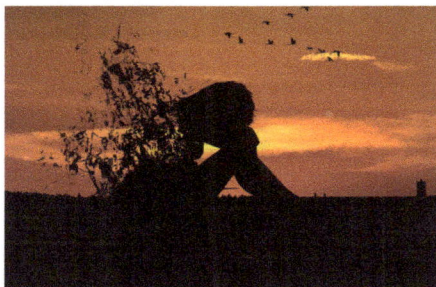

I suck in a deep breath. *Calm*, I tell myself. *It will be okay. Be still and know. Faith.*

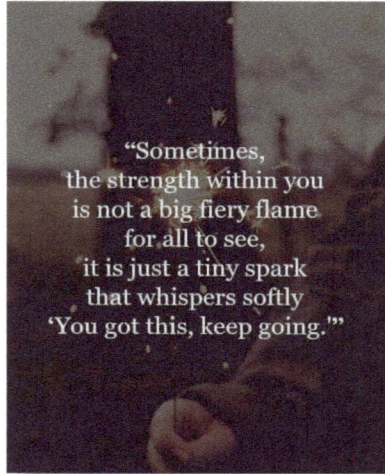

"Sometimes, the strength within you is not a big fiery flame for all to see, it is just a tiny spark that whispers softly 'You got this, keep going.'"

My daughter sits beside me in the waiting room. We're thirty minutes early. I flip mindlessly through one of the 50 million magazines displayed with obsessive spacing. I almost don't want to mess up their perfection.

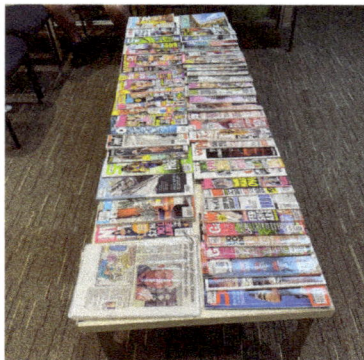

My unfriend, Anxiety, sits beside me and taps me on the arm. I shake my head at it while Tinnitus holds on for dear life. I'm okay. My shadow, Meniere's, is jumping from seat to seat, trying to catch my attention. I ignore it.

Jane greets me with a smile. The universal language that puts you at ease. My unfriend, Anxiety, Tinnitus, Deafness, my shadow, Meniere's, and I follow her to her office.

We sit with a sigh and Jane turns to me. 'Today is our "final expectations" discussion.'

She tells me it's all about ensuring that I know what I am signing myself up for.

She picks up her blue pen, and starts ticking items off her checklist, questioning me for my understanding of each point:
- Technical aspects
- The cochlear implant manufacturer of my choice – Cochlear or MED-EL? I choose Cochlear – based on conversations with many CI recipients and my Cochlear Implant Surgeon
- Ear fitting
- Care of the outer device of the cochlear implant

She stops talking and looks at me. 'All good so far?'

'Yes,' I answer.

She nods, then pulls out colour samples, like choosing colours for a car.

I gaze down at them and narrow my eyes. Skin colour. Brown. Black. Grey. White.

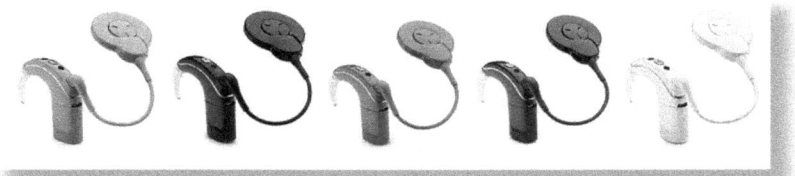

'Which colour would you like?'

I lift my chin a little as I visualise each of them on my head.

'White, please.'

'Really?' Jane looks at my dark wavy hair.

'Yes. Black is the colour of depression. I don't like gray, skin colour or brown. White for me, is a symbol of a new start. New beginnings. Hope.'

'Okay. Just email me if you change your mind,' she says as she takes note of the colour I have chosen.

'Sure,' I say, knowing that I won't be changing my mind.

I am certain the meeting is now over. I have survived yet another appointment. As taxing as they are, the appointments are important. I feel like they are preparing my mind for the change that is to come.

Jane moves her chair backward and stands. 'I'll be back in a moment.' She leaves the room.

I look on the desk at the cochlear implant that will be inserted under my scalp, a hole drilled in my skull, and the electrodes fed inside my cochlear, and am struck with intense panic, my mind saying, 'What are you doing? **What. Are. You. Doing?**'

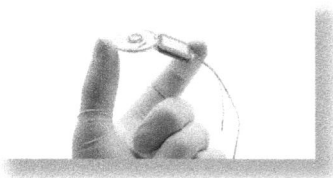

I am filled with an incredible doubt that nearly cripples me.

Do I really need a CI? My shadow, Meniere's, is climbing the large glass windows like Spiderman, and laughing. Tinnitus turns up the volume on a new noise, louder than the rest, and Anxiety is growing exponentially large.

I close my eyes and focus on my good ear. Yes. It feels different. I am losing my hearing in my good ear. The cochlear implant is the right choice.

Jane returns with some paperwork. I quickly switch into a cool, calm, composed mode after my intense moment of panic.

'I need to let you know that if you were going through the public health system, you wouldn't be a candidate for a cochlear implant, as your hearing in you right ear isn't bad enough.'

My eyes widen for a moment. I feel like I am cheating the system with my private health insurance. *What am I doing?*

'I need to talk to you about the bad things about the cochlear implant.

There's bad things? I think.

'Any residual hearing that is left in your left ear may no longer function.'

I frown. 'But I can't hear anything out of it. So, don't the benefits outweigh that risk?'

Jane nods and smiles at me, then says, 'For some recipients, their tinnitus gets worse.'

I nod. *Can this really be true?* My five noises of impossibly loud tinnitus, louder than anything in my life, no matter what my environment is, couldn't get worse, could it? My unfriend, Tinnitus, screams and shouts while doing the happy hoola dance. I flick it a backhand and it behaves.

Jane gives me a smile. 'You are the person with the longest time of deafness to go through our clinic with activation.' She seems kinda excited by that.

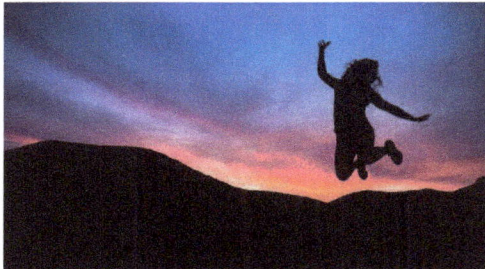

Great, I think. 'I always like a challenge,' I say. I change the subject. 'The technology of the CI blows my mind. It's such a great age to live in. A friend of mine lost his eye while surfboarding and told me that sight for the blind is being developed based on the cochlear technology.'

Jane smiles and nods her head. 'There are companies working on a vestibular type of device for vertigo, based on the cochlear implant technology as well.'

A vestibular pacemaker, I think. My skin prickles. Happiness for my fellow Menierian's and other vertigo sufferers fills me until I overflow with joy. I can't imagine a world without vertigo. But maybe it is getting closer.

Jane looks around her desk at her paperwork. 'Okay – your surgery date is the 19th of December, and switch on of your cochlear implant is the 7th of January. I will organise for delivery of the cochlear implant to your surgeon and then everything is good to go. Any questions?'

I sit for a moment in silence. My shadow, Meniere's, Anxiety, Tinnitus all fold their arms and look at me. Deafness has no idea what is going on. 'You have covered everything exceptionally well. I don't have any questions.'

We both stand and leave the room. *This is really happening.*

Claire smiles at me when I enter the reception room. We walk to the car and she tells me a story about an old lady who kept staring at her. The old lady finally spoke up. 'What are you doing on your phone?'

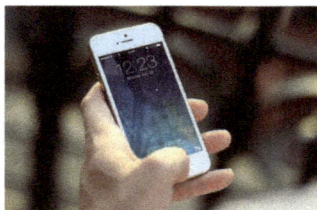

'I'm reading the news,' Claire had said.

The old lady nodded and said to Claire, 'I was on a bus with my friend. We were the only ones without phones. The bus driver said over the speaker, "If you don't put away your phones, I am going to pull the bus over and stop".'

Claire said to me, 'I find that hard to believe.'

We laughed, and then I remembered my very first mobile phone.

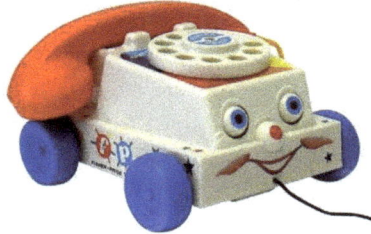

This was my first Mobile phone

Next appointment: *Wednesday, 27th November – balance rehabilitation*

Meniere's disease is ...
violent

Gram dropped to the floor with a loud thud.

I screamed. My breath trembled like an aftershock and I ran through the flower store and around the workbench.

Gram was lying on her back, staring at the ceiling. She swallowed hard and then her chin began to quiver. A tear rolled down the side of her face and disappeared into her hair. 'I hate Meniere's disease!' she said between clenched teeth. 'I feel like I've been cursed!'

I knelt beside Gram. 'Are you spinning? Is it the vertigo?'

'No. It's another symptom of this despicable disease—a drop attack ... I am so filled with the ugliness of hatred, and I don't know who or what to hate. Do I hate me, fallen man, or the disease itself?'

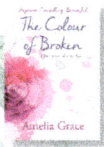

Wednesday 27th November, 2019
balance rehabilitation

Balance

noun: balance; plural noun: balances
1. an even distribution of weight enabling someone or something to remain upright and steady.

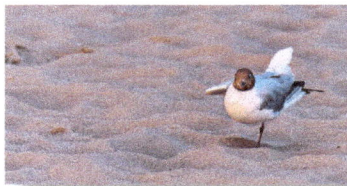

In 2004, nine years after my Meniere's started, I made a conscious decision to have my balance cells destroyed. I couldn't do the horrendous, unpredictable, debilitating, violent, torturous, four-five hours of insane vertiginous spinning and nausea and vomiting and staring at one focus spot on the wall for the entire four-five hours anymore. I was more than done. I didn't want to be here anymore. So when my ENT offered to inject gentamicin into my middle ear to kill off the balance cells, halting the vertigo, I didn't think twice.

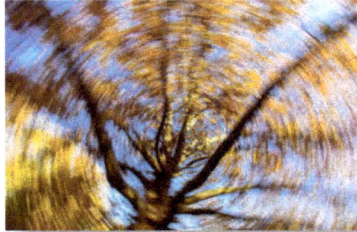

Was the gentamicin my first port of call? Absolutely not. I had already had Meniere's disease for nine years and tried:

* Low salt diet
* Diet elimination
* Stemetil
* Diuretic
* Serc
* Sound therapy
* Acupuncture
* Prednisone
* Grommet

Gentamicin was next. If that didn't work, I was going to have a Vestibular Nerve Section. The gentamicin worked - an answered prayer. One full strength shot injected in through my grommet with some bicarbonate of soda and sterile water mixed with it to make it penetrate better.

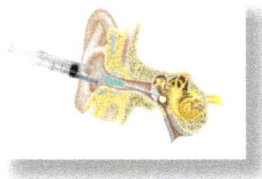

Image: Polyclinique Centre-Ville

The procedure took place at my ENT's procedure room in the city. Before injecting the gentamicin, he spoke to Professor Bill Gibson, the MD guru, in Sydney. I lied on my right side while he injected the concoction in through my grommet in my left ear.

'Isn't that hurting?' he had asked me as he infused the mixture into my middle ear.

'Yes,' I had said, 'but I am envisaging it destroying the Meniere's in my middle ear. It's a mind visualisation technique I taught myself when I was young, when I had growing pains in my knees.'

I remained on my right side, left ear facing the ceiling for 20 minutes after the procedure, then went home, where I went to bed and rolled onto my right side to keep my left ear up. I slept for two hours.

The next day I had bouncy vision when I walked. It has a term – oscillopsia. Oscillopsia is a vision problem in which objects seem to jump, jiggle, or vibrate when they're actually still. It stems from a problem with the alignment of your eyes, or with the systems in your brain and inner ears that control your body alignment and balance. It was a side effect of having my balance cells destroyed. It was a good sign that the gentamicin was working, my ENT had said.

Three weeks later I was back teaching full-time, learning to trust that I wouldn't have anymore vertigo attacks. Since 2004, I have been vertigo free. So thankful for God's mercy and grace.

Choosing to destroy my balance cells to stop the vertigo was not a hard decision for me. Meniere's disease had total control on my life, and I wanted it back. There was a risk of losing all of my hearing, but that was a preferred choice compared to continual suffering through the torturous vertigo. The gentamicin stopped the vertigo. I gained quality of my life again – socialising, working, independence, driving, and slowly became more confident in my life.

I lost a little of my hearing, but not a lot.

If my vertigo returned, would I do it again? *Yes.* But that is also dependent on what new solutions for vertigo are around in the future.

When I joined global Meniere's groups, years later, I discovered that others who had this procedure done were having balance therapy. I was shocked that there was even a thing called balance therapy. When I had my procedure done in 2004, balance therapy didn't exist where I lived. I had to relearn to walk again, finding my new balance, learning my limitations as I went. No help.

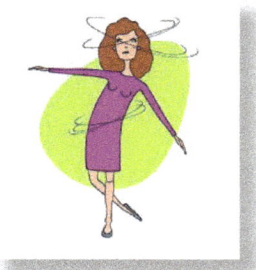

Today, I sit in the reception of the vestibular therapist's office, with a referral from my cochlear implant surgeon.

Mandy greets me with a smile. The universal language that puts you at ease. Curiosity, my unfriends Anxiety, Tinnitus, Deafness, my shadow, Meniere's, and I follow her to her office. I sit on a chair and she questions me about my Meniere's history, writing notes.

'I'm concerned about your imbalance after 15 years. You should not have that deficit anymore. It may point to another problem you have. Do you have Meniere's in your right ear,' she asks.

'No,' I say. My unfriend, Anxiety, stands up.

She frowns at me. 'Let's do some tests and see what is going on.'

She asks me to balance with my eyes closed for 30 seconds. It's a long 30 seconds. I pass this test.

She asks me to walk across the room, heel to toe, heel to toe, heel to toe. I fail miserably. Two steps and I fall over.

Then she asks me to look at the letter "N" on the wall, and moves my head left to right over and over and over, quickly, then asks me whether the letter moves. *Yes.* She repeats that test, but puts her hand on my head and moves my head up and down over and over and over, quickly, asking whether the letter "N" moves. *Yes.* I so hate this. The nausea.

Mandy sits close to me on my left side. I have to sit at a 45-degree angle to her and focus on her nose. She then puts her hand on my head and moves my head left to right over and over and over again, quickly. *Oh the nausea.*

'That's not too bad,' she says.

She repeats the test, but this time she sits on my right side. I try to keep my focus on her nose as she moves my head left to right over and over and over again, quickly. I can not keep my focus on her nose at all.

'Yes. That's the gentamicin damage in your left ear,' she says.

I sit on a massage table.

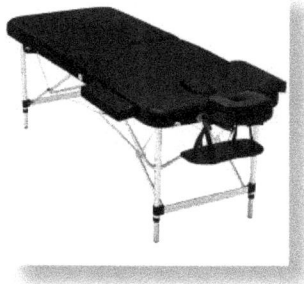

Mandy places some goggles over my eyes. She wants to see if I have Benign Paroxysmal Positional Vertigo (BPPV). She does the Epley manoeuvre. No vertigo or eye movement evident.

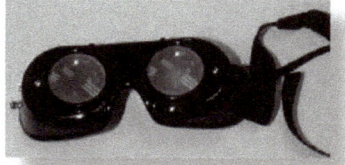

Mandy stands and talks me through some vestibular exercises for neuro-plasticity – the brain relearning balance. I cannot express how happy I am to get these exercises. They will help me no end.

Except, each of the exercises make me feel insanely nauseous. I blow a controlled breath through my lips. I'm an expert at it.

'Do you want to stop?' she asks me during each exercise.

'No,' I say. 'I can do this.' And I get through to the end.

'Can I take Stemetil when I feel nauseous with the exercises?' I ask.

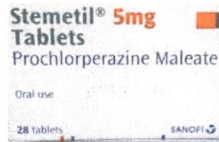

'No,' she says. 'It's a vestibular suppressant, and your brain won't learn the new balance pathways and desensitisation.'

'What about Serc?' I ask.

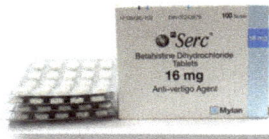

'No. Don't take Serc either,' she says.

'But it is only supposed to increase the blood flow in the inner ear,' I say.

She shook her head. 'No. That's what they want you to believe. It a vestibular suppressant, like Stemetil – it's good for Meniere's, but not other vestibular conditions.'

'Some doctors state it does nothing for Meniere's,' I say, frowning, recalling how my own ENT and the cochlear implant ENT scoffed when I mentioned Serc. I wondered why the makers of Serc would say it increases blood flow, while the vestibular therapist, who specialises in vestibular retraining says it's a suppressant. I know for a fact that many Meniere's people say Serc keeps their vertigo at bay.

'From the conferences I have attended, it does indeed work for many Meniere's patients, not all though,' she adds.

Yeah, I was one who it didn't work for, I think.

I leave her vestibular therapy room, which is in a really old house that is not level. I almost fall over as I walk through it. My shadow, Meniere's, laughs at me. I am armed with vestibular exercises, and an appointment for next week.

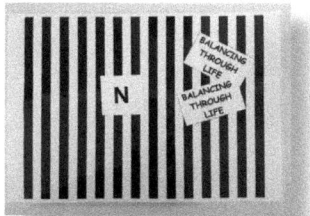

I have now completed all of my necessary cochlear implant work-up appointments.

Next appointment - *the cochlear implant. December 19th.*

Meniere's disease is ...
life destroying

'I hate this. I so, so hate this!' She lifted her face to the ceiling, her eyes closed, tears rolling down her cheeks. She placed a shaky hand on her forehead. 'I'm at the mercy of this disease. I have no control over it and it does what it likes, mocking me in the process.'

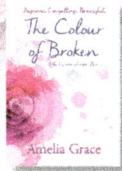

The Colour
of Broken

Amelia Grace

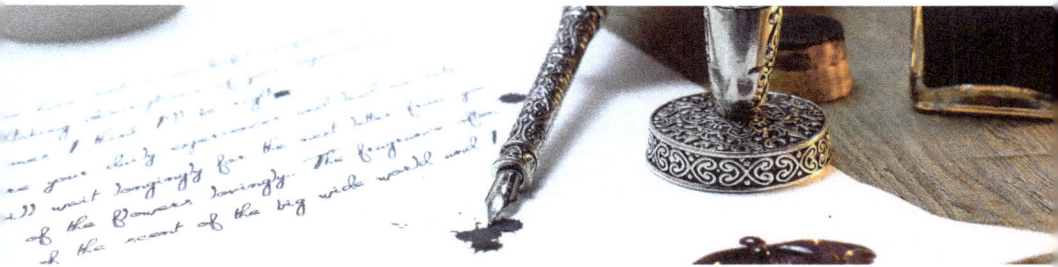

Love Letter To My Left Ear

To My One and Only, Dearest Left Ear,

I know you tried to keep our hearing. I know you tried so hard for so long. You battled against the Meniere's beast with reckless abandon. You fought hard against the inhumane, vicious, violent, vertigo attacks. Together we struggled. Together we cried beyond a thousand tears filled with hope, asking for mercy, until we had no more tears to collect in our bottle of deep sadness, of stolen dreams, of a normal life to live.

'Why?' we asked. 'Why us? Why anybody?' But there were no answers.

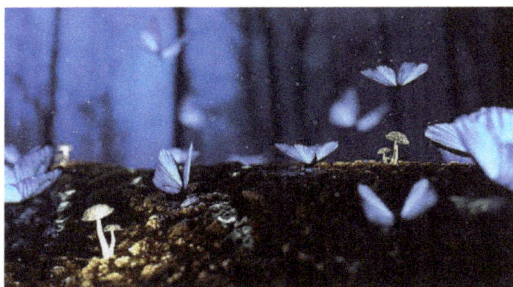

Our world of hearing became muted, little by little. Stolen under stealth within vertigo attacks, leaving nothing but the impossibly incessant loud tinnitus as the flat line of hearing loss took hold – a confirmation of deafness – my brain desperately searching for some sort of hearing, but finding none, so instead, it made up its own sounds; a symphony of incessant annoying pitches, squeals, drones, beeps, cicadas, bees, waveless oceans, electrostatic buzzes, louder than anything I could hear with my remaining hearing ear.

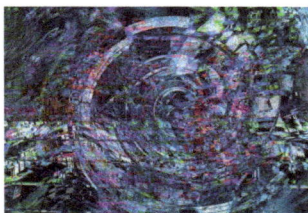

Dear Left Ear, I acknowledge that you bravely and fiercely battled the Meniere's monster since 1995, with all of your might. It was an internal battle unseen against the oppressive, invisible, incurable illness of Meniere's disease. But it wore you down, until you had no more to give. And I thank you for your huge effort in fighting for us.

I heard it too, when the audiologist said in 2019, that we had little to no hearing, then called you a "dead" ear. My hand gently touched you and traced your outline after that blow to the heart.

"Dead". It's such a final word. Complete. Absolute.

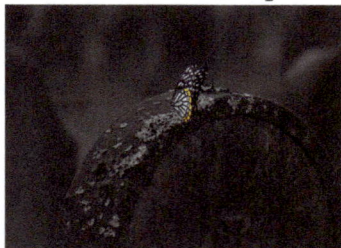

"It's not dead, just dormant!" I wanted to yell. But I didn't, as my heart cracked, the brutal sting of that word "dead", cutting so deeply I wanted to cry. Yet, it made me realise how much I loved you, even though we had been to the deepest, darkest pit of depression together, grappling for hope, desperately searching for a cure for Meniere's disease so I could have you back with your miracle of hearing, so profound and miraculous.

Meniere's disease. The cruel and unforgiving Meniere's disease. It takes and never gives back…

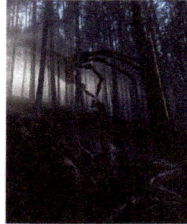

Dear Left Ear, we are rising against the Meniere's monster with a vengeance. No longer will we live our life in submission to the incurable illness. It may be incurable, for now, but we can take a stand. We can take action. We are going to take control of our life. *Our life.* We won't let Meniere's decide our path for us and continue to beat us while we are down.

This is war!

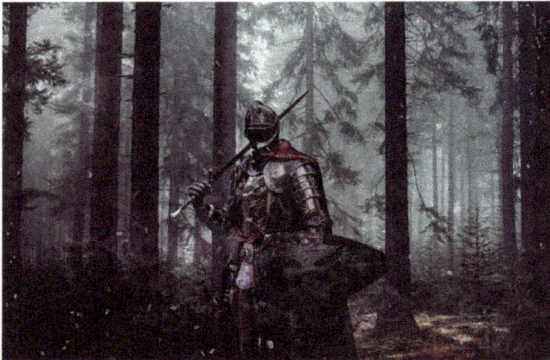

Dear Left Ear, together, we will take back what is ours. We will no longer have vertigo. We will be able to hear again. We will resuscitate your heart of hearing, and tinnitus will be drowned out with sounds of voices, music, and the harmonies of nature.

The battle line is drawn. Our swords unsheathed.

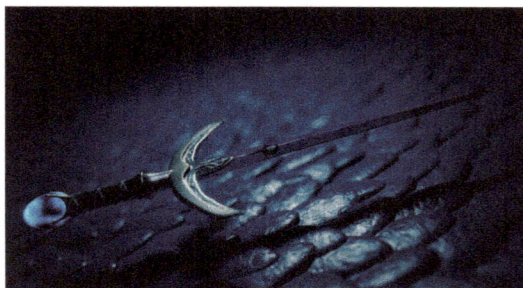

The Meniere's Beast's Weapon – 10 years of violent abhorrent vertigo.

My Weapon – Balance cells destroyed in 2004 by gentamicin, to stop the vertigo (after many other attempts using natural products, acupuncture, sound therapy, medications and medical procedures etc), then vestibular rehabilitation – *battle won.*

The Meniere's Beast's Weapon – Hearing loss and tinnitus.

My Weapon – cochlear implant to restore hearing and eliminate tinnitus.

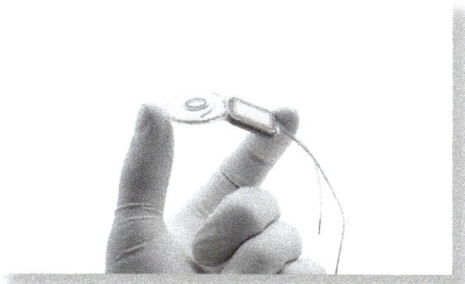

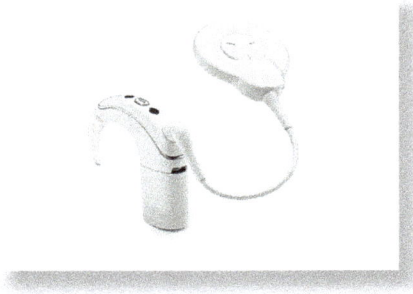

Let the hearing battle begin!

Dear Left Ear, let's do this.

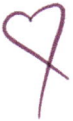

With love,

Julieann

P.S. *We must never forget the medical practitioners who have helped us on this journey. Without their care, compassion and expertise, we would not even be able to enter the battle arena.*

P.P.S. *We must never forget our friends and family who have supported us on this journey. Without them, we would not be able to enter the battle arena.*

Meniere's disease is ...
life changing

Why couldn't the vertigo be stopped? Surely there was a magic pill she could swallow to return her to her normal self? I looked down at my steel-capped boots—my personal protection from a physical attack. But what was there to protect a person from an attack from the inside—from your own body, or your own mind?

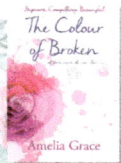

The Colour of Broken

Amelia Grace

Monday December 16th, 2019
three days before the cochlear implant surgery …

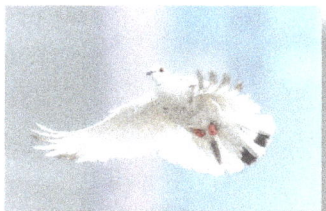

I am engulfed by the feeling of peace. It is flowing through me, around me.

I should be happy. But this sense, three days away from my cochlear implant surgery worries me. It confuses me. Where has my unfriend, Anxiety, gone?

My shadow, Meniere's, looks at me and shrugs.

Some people say anxiety is an illness. A mental health condition. A disorder. A disability. But I have *never* seen it that way. Anxiety, for me, is a super ability. It allows me to look at a situation and see every possible scenario where something could go wrong, and allows me to have a plan in place in my head to react if something does go wrong, even when anxiety is paralysing and jumps out of nowhere while you try to work out what triggered it, going through the motions of a panic attack. It can be so irrational.

In fact, I feel so peaceful, that the reality that I am having surgery to insert technology into my head does not phase me at all. It's surreal, like a dream that will not happen. It's no threat to my being. However, it is so disturbing, that again I am questioning whether I should be getting a cochlear implant. I am okay with hearing with one ear, aren't I? I don't in fact need a cochlear implant. My life is floating along on calm waters …

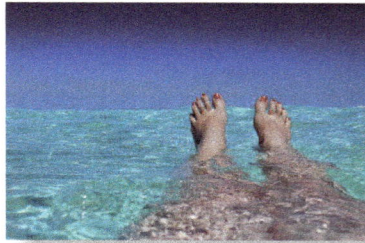

What has changed?

In the middle of the year I was hit with the truth that I was losing hearing in my good ear. I had been living in denial of the results of a hearing test two years prior. I was struggling to hear students at school, and constantly on high alert using my vision to pick up on any nuances, facial expressions, and non-verbal behaviours that would tell me that I had misheard and misunderstood. This combination sent me into a downward spiral with a decision made in an instant to get a cochlear implant. I needed to have some sort of hearing in my future.

But now, I am on school holidays. I happily disappear into my imagination all the time where I never have to rely on my hearing. I am having one-on-one conversations with my family, facing them, and their voices are not competing with background noise.

Life is good.

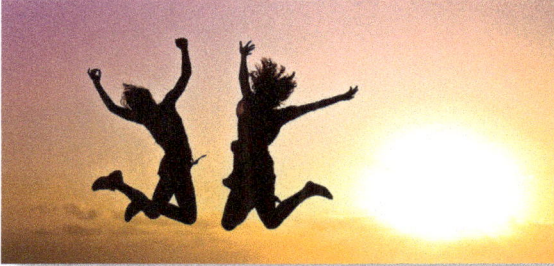

Meniere's disease is ...
isolating

'I don't socialize anymore. I can't hear anyone properly ... in restaurants, or group gatherings, or parties. All I can hear is the murmur of voices. I can't tell what the heck they are talking about and I can see they get tired of me saying "sorry—can you say it again". It's always an imposition for them to repeat it, and then they end up saying, "it doesn't matter", when it does matter—*it does matter to me!* I want to know what they said, it's important to me. All I do now if I do go out, is smile and nod, without knowing what they're saying. And do you know how stupid I look when they're talking about something bad or sad, and I'm smiling and nodding—I feel like the biggest idiot!'

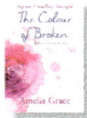

The Colour
of Broken

Amelia Grace

Wednesday December 18th, 2019
one day before the cochlear implant surgery...

I leave the house with a bounce in my step, my shadow, Meniere's, follows closely behind. I am meeting two dear friends for lunch.

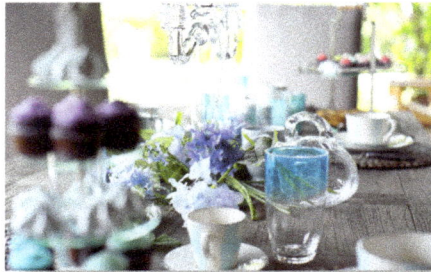

The moment we see each other we smile. The universal language that puts you at ease. I sit at a rectangular table, a friend on either side with me.

My shadow, Meniere's, sits opposite me with a smirk on his face, knowing that I have sat in the wrong place, and I won't be able to hear my friend on the left. I glare at my shadow, Meniere's.

He is not always right!

After 5 minutes, I ask my friend on my left to change seats with me so I can hear better. As I stand, I scowl at my shadow, Meniere's. He is always right. And I am always stubborn.

Halfway through our lunch, I sit back. I have mental fatigue from trying to hear our conversations; from reading facial cues, lips, and gestures, but not well enough the hear the conversation with 100% confidence.

My friend's voices are in competition with loud background noises, and my even louder tinnitus. My deafness is winning.

Two times, a waiter has appeared on my left, and I had no idea that he was standing there asking me a question. By the third time, my friend told me he was approaching so I was aware.

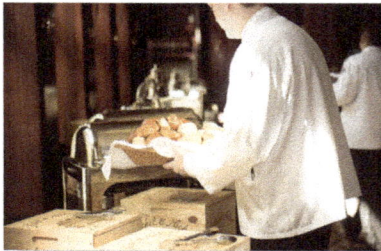

I feel like I am on the outside.

A spectator.

I withdraw inside myself a little and sigh, but stay actively engaged in what conversation I can hear, and join the conversation only when I am 100% confident I have understood what they are talking about.

There is no doubt. I do need a cochlear implant. Without it, I will continue on the spiral to being a social recluse, watching life go by.

Thank goodness for the perfect timing of friends. Without that lunch with my two dear friends, I would have been left forever wondering whether getting a cochlear implant was the right thing to do.

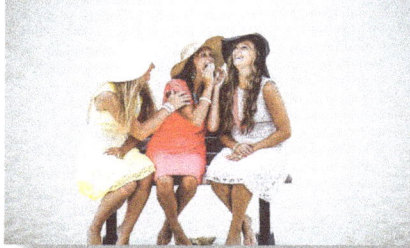

Next … *surgery day.*

Meniere's disease is ...
unforgiving

'I see them ...' she whispered into my ear, 'those suffering like me ... and I want to be the one to stop it for them. Nobody deserves this ... this ... manic, violent, debilitating, depressing, disgusting, deplorable, despicable, devastating, damaging, distressing, diabolical monster of a disease that makes you vulnerable and defenseless. It takes everything, *everything*, Landi, and never gives back ... it takes *everything*.' Gram's voice was tainted with a restrained anger.

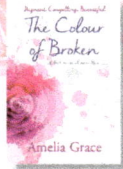

The Colour
of Broken

Amelia Grace

Thursday December 19th, 2019
surgery day ...

The birdsong of the new day wakes me. If I had been sleeping on my good ear, I would never had heard it.

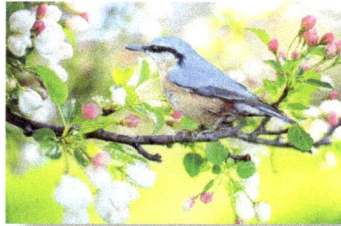

I'm thankful for that precious moment. It's been my survival mantra since battling the ferocious Meniere's disease. *Look for the small things that make me happy, no matter how small or insignificant to others.* It's been 24 years of Meniere's disease now. And it's been a helluva journey that had me on my knees pleading for mercy many times as I battled the violent, abhorrent vertigo that left me a shadow of myself, lost in the darkness of depression, trying to find me, my old happy, carefree, confident, successful self. Menierians know exactly what I am talking about.

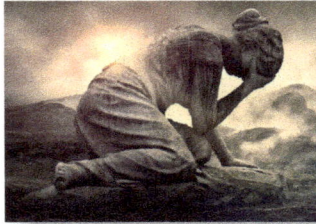

I blink away my past. Today's the day.

The surgical step in regaining my hearing, I think. *There's no turning back. Yesterday was proof, more than enough, that I need the cochlear implant.*

I climb out of bed and walk to the window and look out. There is still smoke haze hanging about from the 100s of fires that have been burning, many of them lit by people who think lighting fires is a fun thing to do. How dare they? I shake my head. We desperately need rain.

I change my focus. I need to finish breakfast by 7:30am and then fast for surgery. Mentally, I tick off what I have already done for today:

* Organised my daughter to spend the day with her father (my husband), to make sure he is okay while I am having surgery. He gets a terrible look of worry on his face, filled with sorrow, when we talk about the possibility of me having vertigo again. It breaks my heart. It's a stark reminder that Meniere's has a powerful impact on those who are spectators to what we go through with this horrid disease.

* Organised for my mum to catch a lift with us to the hospital.

* Organised for my two sons to pick up my dad to come and visit me after the surgery.

* Laughed at the absurdity of all the organisation I must do

to ensure that the wheels turn smoothly.

Time for me.

* Breakfast before 7:30, then fasting. Toast and tea and chocolate.

* Pack the overnight-stay bag for hospital.

* Race to Target to buy some slippers for hospital. I have never owned any. I choose the bunny slippers because I have always wanted to have a rabbit as a pet. In Queensland, Australia, where I live, it's a $44,000 fine if you are caught with a rabbit. This is the closest I can get.

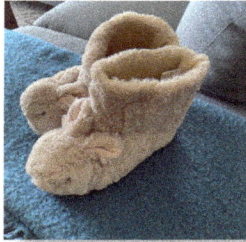

* Double check paperwork.

I still for a moment. *Vertigo.* I have a terrifying fear that it would be awakened by the procedure.

My shadow, Meniere's, is dancing around me smiling. I raise an eyebrow at it and it stops.

The clock ticks over to 10am. It's time to go. It's time to start a new chapter in my Meniere's journey.

I hug each of my sons and tell them that I love them. My eldest son tells me he loves me, and I hear it easily. My youngest son says something after I tell him I love him. In true Meniere's deaf ear fashion, and one sided hearing, I can't hear what he said and say my usual, 'I didn't hear you, can you say it again?' and he says with more volume and clarity, 'I love you, too.'

My heart melts.

I do a final swoop of the house. It is clean and tidy. Then walk to the front door.

My husband has my hospital backpack slung over his shoulder, and my daughter, her heart more beautiful than sunshine, stands beside him. They watch me, worry etched on their faces.

I suck in a deep breath, controlling the deep emotion that tries to surface, not for me, but them. I don't want them to worry.

'I have an amazing feeling of peace. No anxiety at all,' I tell them. And it's the truth.

The front door closes with a faint click. It's symbolic in a way. One door closes, another opens …

I walk to the car thinking, *Anxiety, where are you? My shadow, Meniere's, Deafness and me, are going in for surgery. Where have you gone?* I can't get over the feeling of peace that envelopes me. I decide to accept it and receive this gift from my faith, my heavenly Father, with a full and thankful heart.

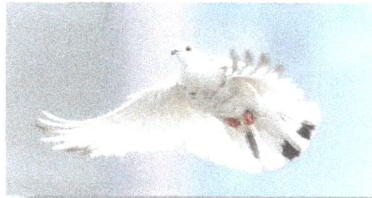

Our car pulls into my parents' house. Mum and Dad greet me with a smile. The universal language that puts you at ease.

'Feeling nervous?' my dad asks, making his hand shake for effect.

'No. Not at all,' I answer. Dad raises his eyebrows at me in disbelief.

'I'm nervous for you,' my mum chips in.

'Good on you, Mum,' I say, offering her a smile.

I hug Dad. Mum sits in the car beside Claire, then I sit in the front seat, and we're off. I'd love to listen to some music with my good ear in the car, but Mum chatters on. I'm guessing it's her nervousness.

We arrive at the hospital and check in, then proceed to the surgery waiting lounge. My family and I take a seat together, while my shadow, Meniere's, bounces on the empty seats. I shake my head at it. Tinnitus is blaring loudly while Deafness looks around. I look for my unfriend, Anxiety, but he's still not here.

It's 11:30am. There's quite a few adults and three children awaiting surgery, and a few of their partners and family members. I watch a man entertain his daughter with a Christmas Elf plush toy. I decide that he is more amused by what he is doing than his child.

My shadow, Meniere's, is sitting on the floor in front of him, watching.

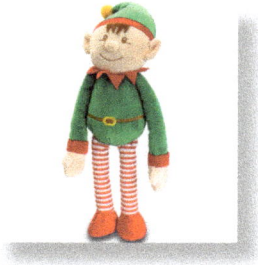

At 12 pm, I'm called to a room by a nurse. She does the pre-op check – temperature, blood pressure, a million questions relating to my health. She tells me that my surgery is scheduled for 2pm, and I return to the waiting room.

At 1:15pm, my anaesthetist appears. I know what he looks like because I Googled his name a couple of weeks ago. My husband and I follow him to a room where we sit and wait for him to speak.

He greets me, talking loudly, over-pronouncing every word

like I am totally deaf in both ears. I think of that annoyance profoundly Deaf people have where normal hearing people think the person will hear better if they talk loudly at them.

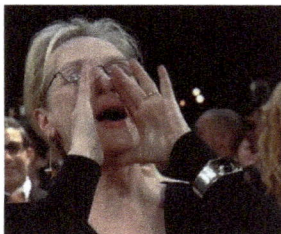

Me: I'm Deaf.
Them:

I tell him I have one good ear and can hear him well. He smiles, and immediately his volume of voice returns to normal.

He asks me medical questions revolving around how I have reacted to anaesthetic with previous operations and takes notes, then I tell him that I have no anxiety about the surgery, and watch for his reaction, both facially and non-verbally with body movement. It still worries me that I'm so peaceful. I am an overthinker after all. I ask him if it is that a thing, like a phenomenon? Or, is there a psychological explanation for it?

He shakes his head and replies, 'It's good not to have anxiety.'

His last words before we exit the room are, 'Don't worry. I'll look after you, I promise.'

We return to the waiting room. I keep looking at my watch, wondering when I will be called in for surgery preparation. It's getting closer to the 2pm surgery time.

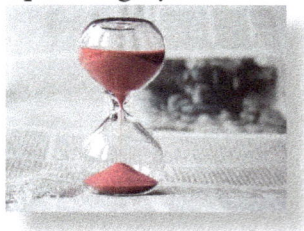

At 1:45pm, I'm greeted by another nurse. It's time to go. I hand out hugs and kisses to my husband, daughter and mother, then disappear, following the nurse to yet another room where she asks me what my name is and my date of birth. She gives me a medical bracelet and cross checks the ID number on it with my paperwork. She shows me the change room, where I am to change into the hospital gown, including covered bare feet and a hospital robe. Once I am dressed, she places tight stockings on my lower legs to prevent blood clots during and after surgery. Then I'm led to a very comfortable recliner chair in another waiting room with a television, where she places a warm blanket over me.

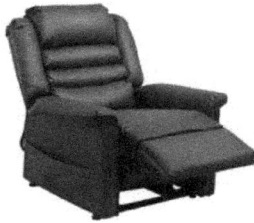

And I wait. But it's a good time for reflection. I think back to the posts from the Cochlear Implant Experiences Facebook group I joined four weeks prior. The discussions and support of other members on there and what I have learned from them has been invaluable.

It is 2:10pm, and I watch other patients come and go. I watch the television, which has closed captioning, then decide to close my eyes for a bit. I hear my name, and I follow another nurse to have a heart trace done (ECG) before returning to the waiting room. Finally, a theatre nurse calls my name, and I follow her to a hospital gurney that will take me to surgery. I don my surgery cap, hair tucked in. I listen to the nurses chatter about holidays they are taking, then my gurney is wheeled to a holding bay. The theatre nurse tells me they need to change around the operating theatre because they will be working on my left ear. She disappears.

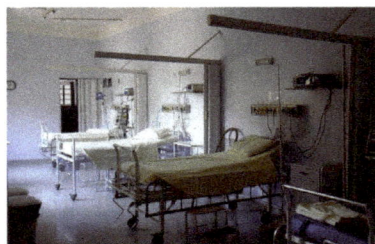

My surgeon enters my holding bay with a smile. He approaches me on my left side, then quickly moves to my right side. 'You will hear me better on this side,' he says. I love him already.

'I need to draw on you to make sure I implant the correct ear. Tell me what surgery you are having done?' he says.

It's a question I have answered many times already, as well as my full name and date of birth. Surgery protocol. 'I'm having a cochlear implant in my left ear,' I answer.

He nods and smiles, then leans over and draws on the left side of my neck, just below my left ear. 'See you soon,' he says, and bounces out of the room with too much energy.

Five minutes later, my theatre nurse is back, and we are travelling the halls of the operating theatres. We enter the surgery room and I gaze around, taking it all in. I see my surgeon studying my MRI, arms folded. He turns and smiles at me. The nurse lines up the gurney to the operating table, and I shuffle over to it, then lie down, ensuring that I am in the middle of the narrow table.

I am surrounded by the anaesthetist, a theatre nurse and my surgeon.

The nurse asks, 'What is the name of your surgeon, and what is your full name and date of birth?'

As I say my surgeon's name I look at him. He has his face mask on, of course. He nods his head and his brown eyes show that he is smiling. I answer the rest of the question and the nurse checks my bracelet ID number to my name.

'What procedure are you having done today?' she asks.

'I am having a cochlear implant in my left ear,' I say.

They all nod.

And then the movement begins. The anaesthetist straightens my right arm and positions it on a support board that juts out from the operating table, then places a tourniquet around my upper arm. He taps my lower arm a couple of times and inserts a cannula. Within 30 seconds I feel myself getting sleepy. The last words I hear are, 'Take a deep breath,' as the anaesthetist places the mask over my face…

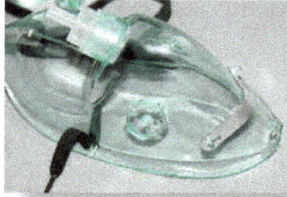

I wake in recovery to the sound of my name being called. I open my eyes and become troubled by what I see. My biggest fear was waking to vertigo, and then having vertigo for days or weeks after surgery.

'I have double vision,' I say to the nurse, then close my eyes. *This isn't right*, I think. *Nowhere in my copious amounts of study and research was double vision mentioned.*

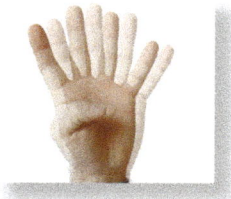

I open my eyes again, and the double vision corrects itself. I feel my body relax after a small moment of panic.

The nurse checks my temperature, blood pressure, oxygen level and heart rate. I keep my eyes open, focussing on any sign of vertigo. None. I then become aware of a tight bandage around my head, over my ear. I have no pain, which, I assume is due to any pain medication given while I was unconscious.

In the next moment, my hospital gurney is moving. I'm being taken to my room for the overnight stay.

As soon as the hospital bed is in position in the room, I look up to see my husband entering, worry painting his face like a fractured mirror. I smile at him, and instantly his worry vanishes, like it has evaporated into thin air.

The nurse fusses about, conducting her observations, recording everything she needs to, and asks if I have any pain, which I don't. My heart rate is sitting at around 58 beats per minute, but that is normal for me.

Then my mum and daughter arrive. My mum smiles slowly, while Claire eyes me warily. She has seen me with too many tears in her lifetime. I smile at them both to put them at ease, but I know they are worried, as their furrowed eyebrows plead for answers to unasked questions.

'I did it,' I say. 'No pain at all. I woke up with double vision. But that's all good now.' I touch the bandage around my head.

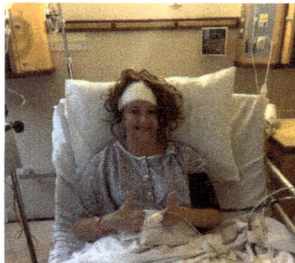

'Nice head band,' my daughter says with a smirk. I grin back at her. She has a way with humour that we both understand. My husband and three children have learned to deal with my Meniere's monster with humour to make me laugh. It's the only way for us all to cope as they watch me fall apart in front of their eyes. They are brave. And observant. And beautiful. This humour from my incurable disease is a bond that holds us together as they gather around me to hold me up from falling in a heap.

I look up as my two sons and my father enter the room. *Well done, boys*, I think, *Grampy would have loved spending time with you in the car.*

Amongst the chatter and explanations and assuring them that I am fine, I discover a tray full of food – chicken soup, a meat dish, vegetables and mashed potato, cake, tea, milk and two bottles of water. Yay! I'm starving! I eat happily, my family tasting this and that as well. The nurse walks in for observations and tells me the surgeon was very happy with the operation. He x-rayed the position of the placement of electrodes while I will still under the general anaesthetic, and that he will be in tomorrow morning to remove the bandages.

After my family leave, I settle in for some much-needed sleep amongst the hospital alarms and beeps.

Still no pain at the surgery site.

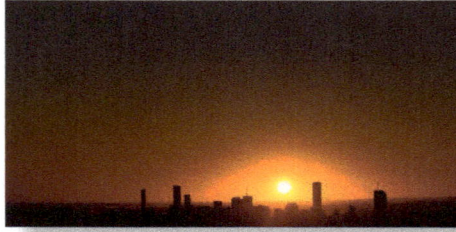

Friday 7am …

My surgeon enters the room with a calming presence.

'How are you?' he asks. His gaze is focussed on my face, waiting for my answer.

'Great,' I say. 'No pain. Did you give me any pain medication during surgery or after?'

He shakes his head.

'I've had no vertigo. Just double vision when I woke in recovery. Are you happy with the surgery?'

'Very,' he says. 'I managed to get the electrodes all the way into your cochlear.'

My eyes widen. I remember the cochlear audiologist telling me that sometimes the surgeon can only get the electrodes partially into the cochlear. 'Wow,' I say. I can't believe it.

He walks to the basin and washes his hands, and takes some scissors from a tray, then walks around to the right side of my bed. 'Let's take the bandage off and see how it looks. I'll have to ruin your great hair style,' he jokes. He uses the surgical scissors and cuts through the bandage and studies the incision site. 'Looks good. Sleep sitting up for a few days and don't wash your hair. No heavy lifting or sneezing. I'll see you on Monday at 10:45am. Any questions?'

'Aaah – no. Just … thank you for looking after me.'

He gives me a nod and a smile. 'Take is easy, and I'll see you Monday.'

10am

My husband arrives. He hands me a copy of my own novel that has a main character with Meniere's disease. It's a gift to the nursing staff. And a gift for those with Meniere's disease. It will help the nursing staff understand what Meniere's is really like – physically, socially, emotionally, psychologically. We need to find a cure! I sign it for them.

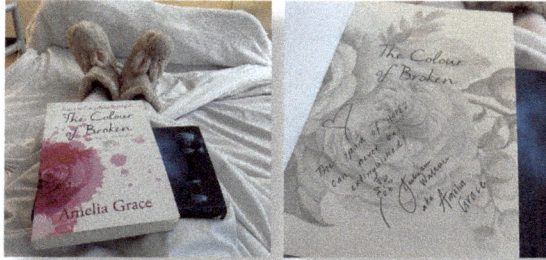

After final observations and cannula removal, I am discharged from the hospital. I am in disbelief at how good I feel. And I am soooo thankful with a heart overflowing with gratitude – my faith, my medical specialists, the nurses, my family – it takes a village.

Life is good. The light shines more brightly when you have struggled through the darkest of dark storms.

Next: *feeling anxious*

Tinnitus is ...
frustrating

I watched as Gram arranged the Japanese magnolias, camellias, kumquats, loropetalum, and bottlebrush—whites, pinks, yellows, dark pink, blues, orange and red—with greenery to set it off, all in a metal goblet vase with handles, humming while she worked. The fragrance of sweet candy flowed around the flowers. It was a breath of loveliness from the magnolias.

'Does your humming add extra love into the creation?' I asked.

'Perhaps ... it's more for me, to try and tune out the incessant loud tinnitus that haunts my ear non-stop. Five noises! It's louder than anything else I can hear, even when I go to a live performance!'

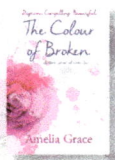

Tuesday January 7th, 2020
anxious

It's two days before my cochlear implant activation and I'm sitting at my desk, writing my new novel, *All the Colours Above*. An overwhelming emotion hits. I want to cry. I want to ugly cry. I catch my sob and swallow the lump in my throat and refocus on my writing, listening to cello music with my right ear, trying in vain to hear over the incessant extra loud tinnitus in my deaf left ear – five different noises. It always wins, even at music concerts. I haven't heard silence for 25 years. Nothing I can listen to masks the sound of tinnitus.

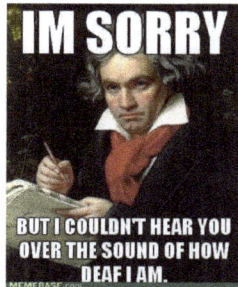

Three years ago, I received a cello as a birthday gift. I wanted to learn to play it so I could hear the music in my memory when all my hearing was gone. I wanted to play it and feel the vibration of the music inside me, so I could burn into my mind how music would make me feel when I could no longer hear. *The emotion of music.* That is why we all love it so much. It makes us feel. *Emotion.* It's what makes us human.

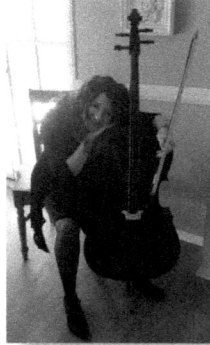

I've been playing the piano since I was eight, and can see the written notes inside my head when music is played. I can look at a sheet of music with no sound, and hear the sound of the inky musical notes on the paper. But it's the cello I love the most.

You never realise how important something is until it is gone. Anyone who has something wrong with their body can vouch for that. Look after yourself. Not that I did anything wrong to lose my hearing. It's Meniere's disease that has done that. I hate it with a passion – not just for me, but what it does to people. I know several people with Meniere's who have taken their lives because of it.

No more. No. More. Enough is enough!

Sometimes, when I am playing music on my computer whilst writing or working, I stop and put my hands on the two speakers on my desk, and place my foot on the sub-woofer on the floor.

I close my eyes and concentrate on the *feel* of the vibration. The vibration of the high and low sounds and everything in between. The light vibration. The strong vibration. The combination of vibrations.

I love it. And hate it.

I would love it because I could still hear it with my "good" ear. I would hate it because I am losing hearing in my "good" ear as well. It would send me into a downward spiral each time, knowing that one day I would never hear music again while walking the earth. Did I do something to cause this? It tortures my mind if I let it. Then I am reminded that my life is all the more richer because of what I have been through.

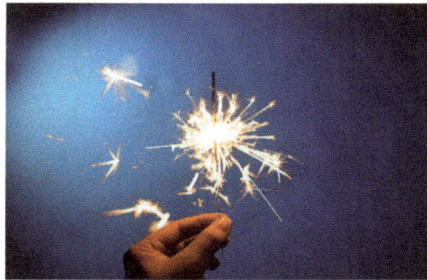

It's the day before activation.

I'm almost going into a panic. *Breathe.* I feel like a bird that has been trapped inside a cage for too long for it to remember freedom, and when the door is opened for it to fly from its prison, it stays there, because it feels safe.

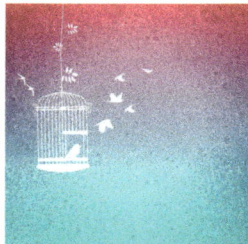

This is me.

A prisoner in my own body.

I've had Meniere's disease for 25 years (2020). Nearly half of my lifetime.

To be honest, there are many days that have been hell.

Friends and family never saw that. They only saw the happy me. The one wearing the mask, fooling the world that I was okay.

I faked being well.

I'm a pro at it. I can't remember what it's like to feel "normal". My life with Meniere's disease is lived within strict limits as to what I can do, what I can eat, choosing to isolate myself from social activities because I can't hear, or I am scared of having a vertigo attack, or the worst one – *rejection* – because of my hearing loss and I can't participate, or because I have answered a question wrongly because I couldn't hear them, and I didn't want to ask them what they had said for the fifth time.

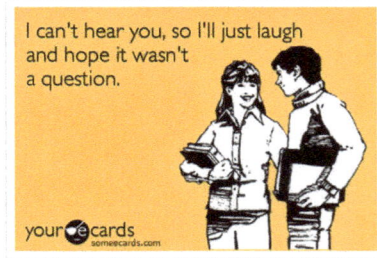

To have no vertigo. No tinnitus. And have hearing in my left ear again … what is that? Is it even possible? What will I become? Will I still be me?

I admit. I am struggling big time. So I keep working on my new novel.

I'm 13,000 words in, and it keeps me from dwelling on the upcoming, perhaps, life changing event tomorrow.

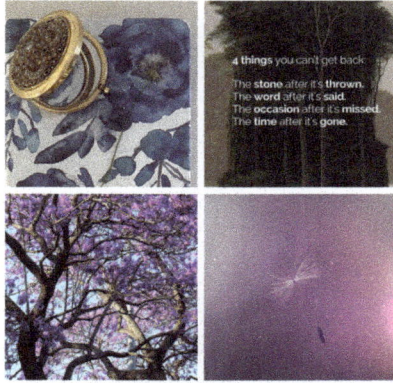

In every cochlear implant group I have joined, the words keep being repeated, "it will change your life".

But how? Is it that I will be able to hear from my left ear again? And that's it. What exactly will it change in my life? Will I like it?

Next appointment: *activation day*

Meniere's disease is ...
isolating

Gram closed her eyes and a tear escaped. She took a slow, deep breath. 'I hate Meniere's disease, Yolande. I hate everything about it! I hate that people can't see what I feel and suffer. I hate that it's an invisible illness. Some of my friends even think I'm faking it! Little do they know I am faking being well ... it's exhausting!' Gram brushed her hands over her face. Her beautiful face. 'It's so exhausting!'

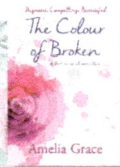

Thursday January 9th, 2020
activation day...

Cochlear implant activated. My mind is blown. My brain is scattered as I write this entry.

A thousand tears of feelings and thoughts, marvelling at technology – invented in Australia. Eternal thanks to you, *Professor Graeme Clark.*

I have warned my family – "Danger. I may break into unpredictable sobbing at any time. Good tears. Very good tears."

I am overwhelmed by feelings of intense happiness. Feelings of release from the Meniere's prison. A thousand memories of my life with Meniere's and what I have been through enter my mind. The vertigo. The abhorrent vertigo of hell that takes your hearing. Your happiness stolen. The darkness of depression that wants to take your last breath.

I feel like I have been freed ...

I can't write anymore today ... I am too overwhelmed with

emotion, and noise, and information. The world is so unbelievably noisy with a cochlear implant.

When the impossible becomes possible.

I am so beyond thankful …

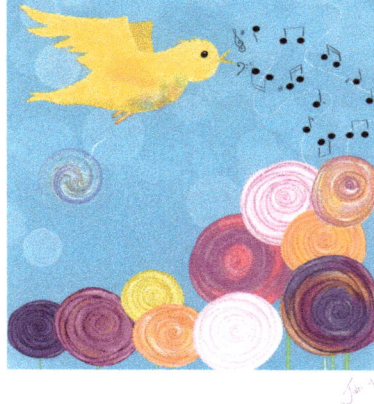

Artwork by Julieann Wallace, 2020

Cochlear Implant Activation, 9th January
it did change my life

The alarm is sounding. It's 6am. But it doesn't wake me, my husband does. I am lying on my "good' hearing ear, so I hear nothing. He touches me to wake me and I struggle to open my eyes. I'm tired. I'm so tired. I haven't slept well because it's hot and humid. Summertime. The night-time low was 24 degrees Celsius.

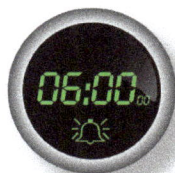

I roll over and vertigo hits me, followed by nausea.

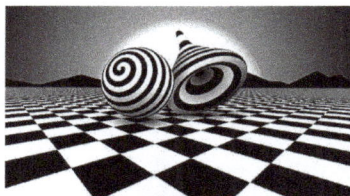

Great, I think, as my world spins. I hold still and the room stops spinning and the nausea goes. *BPPV.* A misalignment of the crystals in the inner ear. I know I can do the Epley Manoeuvre to stop it. But I don't want to do it until I check with my cochlear surgeon in 4 weeks' time.

I breathe a messy breath through my lips and sit up. First, I focus on the wall to check that my world is not spinning again, then stand slowly, to ascertain whether my balance feels okay. I remember it's cochlear implant activation day. But I'm so tired. Activation can't be on a day when I am exhausted before the day begins. It didn't happen that way in my imagination when I looked forward to hearing again.

I sigh.

I push forward with my morning routine. Breakfast is low key. Toast with peanut butter and a cup of tea. My unfriends, Anxiety, Tinnitus and Deafness join my shadow, Meniere's, and me at the table. The five of us together again. I frown. Why do I feel anxious about activation, but not about the two-hour surgery where they drilled a hole in my skull three weeks ago?

I stop before the door before we leave to drive to the city. I feel safe here, behind the closed door. Comfortable. Once I open that door, my world is going to change. I take a deep breathe, place my hand on the doorknob and turn it.

I step out into my future.

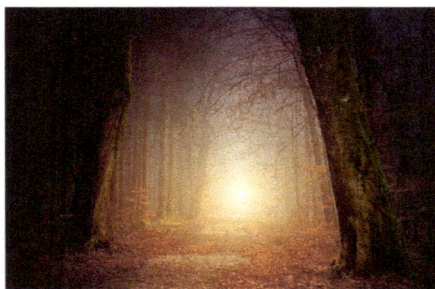

My husband and I arrive early for the appointment. We sit in the waiting room where the perfectly arranged magazines adorn the table, painstakingly presented. When my husband takes a magazine, flips through it and plops it back on the table, I can't help but to straighten it up so it is like the others.

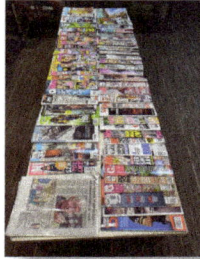

I look up when I think I hear my name called.

Jane, my cochlear audiologist greets me with a smile. The universal language that puts you at ease. Anxiety, Tinnitus, Deafness, My Shadow, Meniere's, my husband, and I follow her to her office. We all sit down, except for my shadow, Meniere's. He's jumping up at the window overlooking the city, and sliding down with a giggle. I shake my head at him.

'Welcome back,' Jane says. 'How did the surgery go?'

'Good,' I say. 'I've had no pain, no major vertigo, just little spins when I roll over. BPPV. I can fix that with the Epley Manoeuvre, but I want to wait until I see my surgeon in a few weeks.'

Jane shakes her head. 'The little spins may not be BPPV. Sometimes drilling the hole in your skull can upset your inner ear and cause that. It will get better.'

Oh. I am surprised by that information. I smile. 'The surgeon managed to get the 22 electrodes all the way in. He was really happy with that,' I say to distract my thoughts that I may have vertigo again.

'Wonderful. Plus you have two earth electrodes in there as well.' Immediately my mind turns to the memory of me out in the storm the other day. I had rushed inside in case my implant attracted lightning.

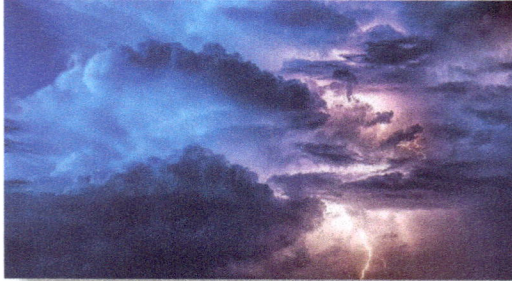

Then, on researching lightning and cochlear implants, I am no more likely to be struck by lightning than anyone else. *Phew!*

Jane turns to my husband and shows him what has been implanted into the cochlear of my inner ear. 'The electrodes are 1/5 of the width of a hair strand, in size.'

My husband's jaw drops to the floor. He shakes his head. It's hard to comprehend.

'Okay. Are you ready for today?' she asks.

I nod, and see Anxiety double his size beside me. I want to grab a pen and stabbed him so he farts all the air out of him. My shadow, Meniere's, sits in the corner and lowers his head. Tinnitus is doing pirouettes in a tutu. My life really is a circus!

Jane places the external hardware over my ear, attaches the transmitting coil to the magnet that sits under my skin on my scalp, all the while explaining how it works. The enthusiasm in her voice tells me how much she loves her job. She is super excited about switching on my cochlear implant.

Once the processor and transmitter are in place, Jane sits on her chair. I'm knotting my fingers together as my skin burns.

I frown. I can't hear a thing in my Meniere's ear. Nothing has changed. My tinnitus is still screaming at me.

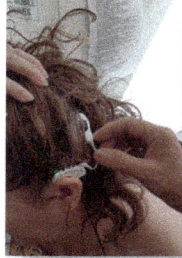

She attaches a wire to the speech processor around my ear and taps a few keys on the computer. She smiles and says all the electrodes are looking good. Then she taps another key and I still. My heart starts to race and my eyes widen. I can hear a few crackles and pops.

'Can you hear this, Julieann?' she asks in her English accented voice.

Three beeps sound in my deaf ear. Then another three at a different pitch, and another three.

'Yes,' I say, my voice cracking. I cover my eyes as tears fall. I can't stop from crying.

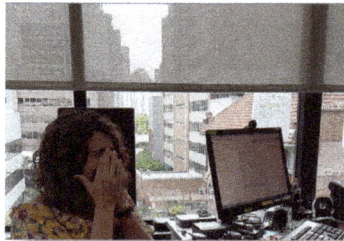

'I can hear that,' I add.

'Good,' she says and smiles. 'Are you okay? There's tissues behind you.'

'Yes,' I squeak. I grab a tissue and look over at my husband.

His eyes are red-rimmed and wet. He has been a part of my journey. 25 years of being a spectator to my incurable Meniere's disease, where he could do absolutely nothing to help me, except clean out the vomit bucket time after time after time after I had vomited violently whilst spinning, or attending the emergency room when I was so dehydrated from vomiting that it was dangerous to my health, or when we thought the violent spinning wouldn't end. We've been married for 31 years. He knows exactly what physical, emotional and psychological toll it has taken on me. He has seen me during my darkest days.

Yet, I spared him from witnessing the darkest of dark days when I no longer wanted to be here, when I wasn't the colour of grey with an "e", nor the colour of gray with an "a", but the colour of black.

From my novel – *The Colour of Broken*

Yolande, the main character is sitting in the chair, talking to her psychologist …

'*What colour are you?*'
I took a deep breath and twisted my fingers together. My stomach tightened. I cleared my throat. 'The colour of broken …'
Dr Jones was silent.
I stopped breathing when anxiety rose inside me like a wall of lava, about to incinerate me. It was freaking me out that she now knew this about me, and that she had not reacted to the description of my colour.
'*And what colour would that be?*' *she finally asked.*
I breathed out through my lips, slowly, steadily, counting to five in my head. 'Gray with an "a".'

'There's a difference?'

'Oh, yes. Grey with an "e" is very different to gray with an "a".'

'How?'

'Grey with an "e" is like the rain clouds. It's melancholy, but an enjoyable melancholy that builds up until it releases, and then it's like petrichor, the smell of the rain after warm, dry weather. Satisfying. Grey with an "e" is also when deep thought, philosophy and ponderings happen. Everyone should experience grey with an "e", it helps to discover parts of you that you never knew existed, and it can vanish without leaving a bitter aftertaste.'

'Tell me about gray with an "a".'

I looked down at my knotted hands. 'Gray with an "a" is ... never enjoyable—it's a very dark gray. It's self-judgement, doom and gloom, forever hanging around and within. It wants to drag you into the dark abyss of the colour black, that absorbs all colours ... the colour of self-condemnation, the colour of depression, the colour of death of the physical body.'

'But not the spiritual body?'

'No.' I didn't want to add any more to this conversation. It was painful to talk about.

'So, me being a supposedly normal person, could I see your gray with an "a"?'

'No. Because I mask it. And my gray with an "a" is not a plain gray with an "a". It's a crackled dark gray, with other colours that seep out ... sometimes.'

'What colours would they be?'

'Drips of red for anger ... specks of black—' for self-hate, '—for my secret, blushes of pink for my love for Mia and my family, and explosions of turquoise that screams at me to love myself ...'

'That's very insightful, Yolande. It's highly intuitive. I'm curious ... when you look at me, what colour am I?'

I hesitated before I spoke. I never told anyone the colour I had appointed to them for fear of them running from me. But Dr Jones, she was different, she would understand …

'You are … magenta,' I finally said. 'It's the colour of a person who helps to construct harmony and balance in life, hope and aspiration for a better world—mentally and emotionally,' I said, and held my breath, waiting for her reaction.

She raised her eyebrows at me. 'That's an amazing gift to have in your mind toolbox, Yolande. Does it ever lie to you?'

Jane my cochlear audiologist says, 'I'm going to switch on each of the electrodes, one by one. Tap on the table when you hear the beeps.'

And so it begins. As I hear beeps, and tap on the table, hope rises in me like a sunflower blooming, facing its sun. I hear 21 out of 22 electrodes. Jane is ecstatic.

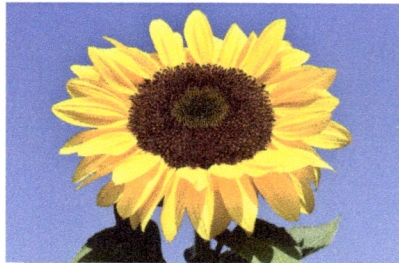

I am in shock and tears trickle down my face. *I can hear!*

Jane looks at me and smiles. 'Do you need a break?'

'No,' I say. I am beyond fascinated. In awe. What an age to live in with medical science, discoveries and inventions.

'Let's try some speech,' she says. She taps a few more keys, and suddenly there are words in my cochlear implanted ear.

I start crying, wiping a thousand tears from my cheeks. 'I can hear what you are saying,' I sob. 'But you sound like you have been inhaling helium!'

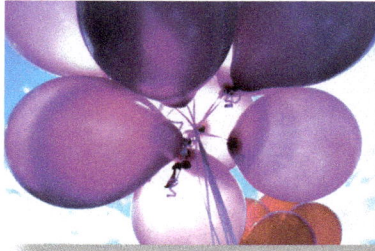

Jane's face lights up with a smile. 'You can! That is so wonderful!' She is looking at me with a contagious joy.

She continues talking. I hear her chipmunk voice, but I can't understand her. She keeps talking, and with my good ear, I hear that she explains that as she keeps talking for another 10 minutes, my brain will start understanding better. She says the hearing part of the left side of my brain has been used for some other processes since I lost my hearing. And now it is shuffling, trying to find my speech and sound memories to make sense of what it is hearing. It is using auditory pathways and memories, and must work at a higher level to pull together the information to have bi-normal hearing. The brain must code all the information coming in.

And then suddenly, like a light has been turned on, I can understand much of what she is saying, as words. Not all of them, but quite a few. For the words I don't get, my mind fills in the blanks with words to match the meaning of what she is saying.

I am speechless.

She turns to my husband. 'Say something to Julieann.'

I look at him and smile.

He smiles back. I see his lips move. I wait for the sound of his chipmunk voice. I swallow and my skin burns. His voice doesn't even register as a chipmunk. I can't hear his voice at all!

His eyes widen in panic.

Jane jumps in quickly in a calm and encouraging voice. 'That's okay. It will happen.'

Jane reaches over and pulls out a foam ear plug and puts it firmly into my good ear. Then she places a hearing muff over my good ear.

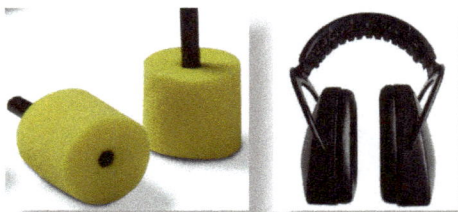

I have lost all hearing that I have been relying on to hear and understand conversation.

Jane continues talking like we are in a normal everyday conversation. I stare at her, trying to get what she is saying. It is so hard. Her voice is sound, but not words.

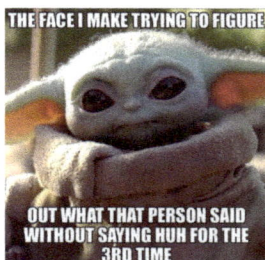

I focus harder, and slowly, some of the sounds become words. She stops and asks me a question. I stare at her blankly. I am trying to figure out what she has asked. I am trying to piece together what words I understood of the question, and with the missing words, I am working on using any visual cues from what she is doing, plus I am trying to read her lips.

Finally, I answer with a smile. 'Yes. I can hear you. And your speech is starting to sound like words.'

'Well done!' she says. And I understand her chipmunk voice perfectly. She then explains about the delay happening in my brain with the speech and understanding. She knows how hard I am working to try and understand the new input into my brain.

'Can you hear this?' she rattles a piece of paper in front of her.

'Yes,' I say, although it doesn't sound like paper, but an unrecognisable noise.

She stands and goes behind me and I hear another noise. I nod my head. I can hear it. She shows me a tissue that she rubbed in her palms. I am absolutely gob-smacked.

She asks me to repeat words. I get most of them right, guessing some of them. Then Jane covers her mouth so I can't read her lips. I hear her, but not clearly enough and get some of the words wrong.

She turns to my husband and asks him to speak to me again, and he does.

I still can't understand him, at all.

She tells him to slow down, and break his sentences into chunks, and not to run the words together.

He tries again.

I smile at him and say, 'No. You don't sound like Darth Vader.' He smiles. He's happy now.

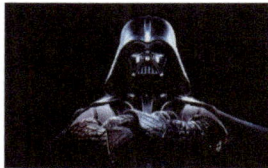

Jane grins. She goes through the Cochlear Australia backpack that is mine to keep. It is filled with bits and pieces for care of my cochlear implant external hardware, plus other bits and pieces and chargers and batteries and paraphernalia. She shows me how to use everything, and then asks me to do the same. It fits in perfectly with my teaching philosophy.

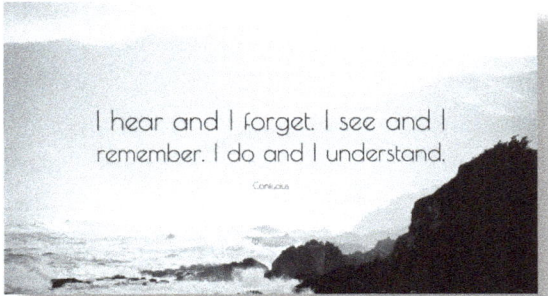

After two hours of intense concentration, she asks in her chipmunk voice, 'Is there anything you want to ask me before you leave today?'

I think for a moment. I've had way too much information overload. My brain is working double time and I am tired. 'Is it okay to wear my new hearing to the Big Bash Cricket game tonight?'

Jane laughs. 'Yes. If you like. It will be very noisy though.'

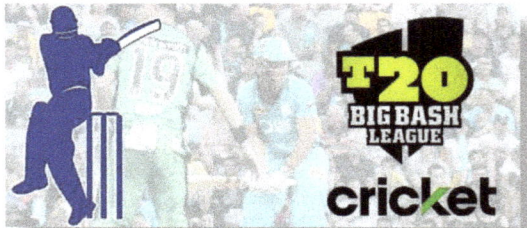

My husband and I leave her office, take the elevator and walk out into the real world. I stop for a moment, wondering if I can hold my emotions together. The impact of activation has been overwhelming. Two hours ago I had walked into Jane's office deaf in one ear. Now I walk out, hearing with two ears.

The thought is profound.

My husband looks at me. 'Are you okay?' His eyebrows are pulled together. For a moment, I wonder how hard this has been on him?

'Yes.' I blink away tears, then start to walk again.

The world is noisy. Terribly noisy. I hear everything in a tinny, echoing, chipmunk way. My brain is detecting two lots of hearing with everything – my deaf, now hearing Meniere's ear, hearing conversations of chipmunk voices, and a chipmunk city noises of its own, while I listen with my good ear to the same thing with normal hearing. The two sides of my brain haven't synced yet. They are acting independently of each other.

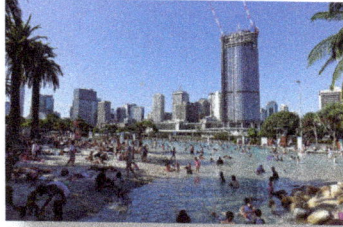

I laugh to myself. How privileged am I to be able to experience this oddity? My heart overflows with gratitude.

I take confident steps into my new normal. Into my future. Bilateral hearing. Something I haven't had for 15 years. Something I thought would be impossible.

Before I go to bed, I remove the external hardware. Immediately my ear feels full and profoundly deaf. My tinnitus returns. But that's okay. That's my other normal. Two of me.

I reflect on my most extraordinary day – five times I have stilled at big moments:

1. When the cochlear implant was activated and I could hear! My mind was blown!

2. When I heard music. I cried so hard my husband wanted to pull over the car to make sure I was okay.

3. I located the direction of a sound. I haven't been able to find where a sound is coming from for 15 years. The ramifications of this for me in the classroom will change my stress level as I teach.

4. I heard a man's lower chipmunk voice while waiting to catch the bus after the cricket …

The cricket … I think back to the Big Bash Cricket and smile. On entry, I was pulled aside for a security check, the metal detector waved over and around me – it always happens to me at airports too. It's become a running joke with my family. I held my breath, wondering whether my cochlear implant would set the detector off. It didn't.

And Jane was right. The Big Bash was very noisy. But it was so worth it. And I'm taking marshmallows to toast in the flames next time!

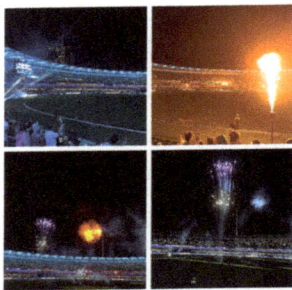

And number 5 … I entered our walk-in wardrobe. As I stood there trying to decide what to wear to the cricket, I froze. Something was wrong. *Very wrong.* My heart raced and I started to panic. I couldn't hear anything. Not even from my "good" ear. I felt for the cochlear implant external hardware. It was still there. I ran my hands over my arms to make sure I was still me, and I wasn't dying – seriously!

Something wasn't right.

I could hear absolutely nothing. *Nothing!* I spoke to check that the cochlear implant was still working. Maybe the power pack had gone flat? I heard my own voice as well as my chipmunk voice. Two of me. I stopped and listened again in the stillness of my walk-in wardrobe.

There was silence.

Utter. Beautiful. Silence. No tinnitus.

Silence after a quarter of a century. I closed my eyes and let my tears fall, covered my mouth and ugly cried. *Silence.*

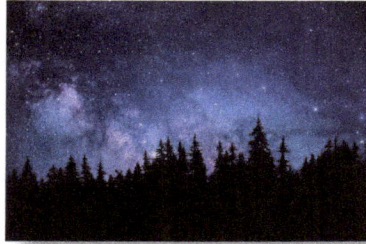

The gift of hearing. I am so beyond thankful. I have no words to explain what it feels like to have the cochlear implant activated and to hear again. My faith. Health professionals. Family. Support of friends and Facebook groups. It takes a tribe.

The cochlear implant has changed my life. On activation. It has made the impossible, possible. Meniere's disease may not be curable, yet, but we can take back from Meniere's what is has taken from us.

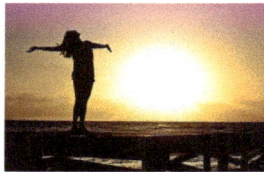

A Cochlear Implant is ...
restoring

I want to hear music again—the singing, the instruments, the bands. I want to hear songs of love, songs of sadness, songs that make me feel high. I want to hear all the instruments in an orchestra—and all the stupid synthesiser music, no matter how ridiculous the sound is. I want to hear voices.

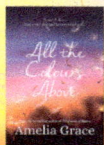

All the Colours About
Amelia Grace

Learning to Hear
mental exhaustion

Fatigue

noun: fatigue; plural noun: fatigues

1. extreme tiredness resulting from mental or physical exertion or illness.

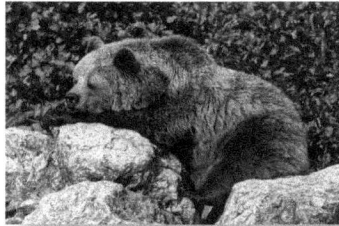

December 19, 2019, I had cochlear implant surgery. On the 9th of January, 2020, my cochlear implant was "activated". My world of deafness, including the five roaring noises of tinnitus changed. I could hear again for the first time in 15 years!

My cochlear audiologist, Jane, warned me, 'You will have mental fatigue from hearing again with your left cochlear.'

Yeah nah, I thought. *I've had the repugnant, revolting, repulsive Meniere's disease for 25 years now, three children and a teaching workload. I know exactly what mental and physical fatigue is like. The simple act of hearing again will leave me fatigued? I doubt it!*
Yeah Nah. Australian slang for no.

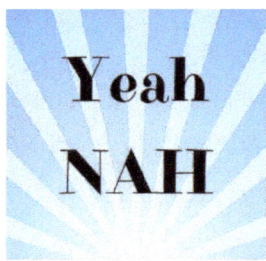

I enter the outside world. *Reality.* I'm no longer safe and comfortable in the confines of the quiet audiologist's office, where Jane's reassuring smiles, encouragement and support, wrap me like a warm blanket on a freezing winter's night.

My eyes widen. It's so NOISY! I hear EVERYTHING! But not the sounds of normal hearing, but of cochlear implant hearing, newly activated: chipmunk voices, robotic representations of every sound my 22 electrodes can feed into my auditory nerve. I am told that the sound I hear now, is not what I will hear as I continue to attend "mapping" sessions. Sounds will become more "normal-ish", like what I hear with my right ear.

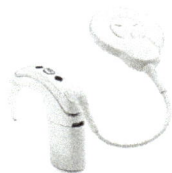

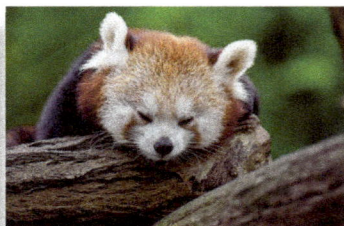

After 10 hours of wearing my processor, I am fatigued. I feel like a flat battery.

Nah Yeah. Yes. Jane was right. *Again.*

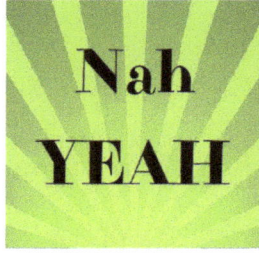

My cochlear audiologist explained, 'It's like you're a baby again. You hear absolutely everything. For your left hearing centre in your brain, every noise is new, and it's working hard to work out whether to file the sound as an important sound, or background sound that it doesn't have to pay attention to. And the two hemispheres of your brain are not working together, yet. But they will.'

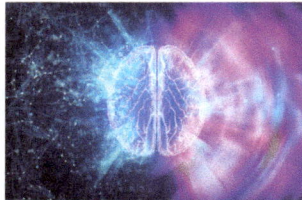

She continued. 'When you lost your hearing 15 years ago, your brain re-used that area for something else, and now that it is stimulated again with hearing, your brain is madly re-organising what parts of your brain are used for what. It is also accessing your auditory memories to match up to what you are hearing now.'

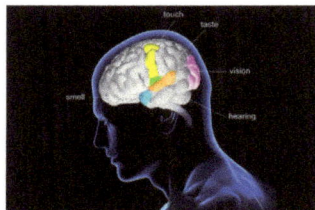

WOW! Mind blown.

Not only by the fact that I can hear again, but by the knowledge that the brain has a design and intelligence that is beyond human understanding.

My cochlear implant journey has been a road filled with new learnings, revelations and knowledge. My erudite self is soaking up anything and everything about hearing, the cochlear and the brain.

The more I learn, the more I realise what an amazing piece of architecture our brain is, one that cannot be replicated. It's complexity and control of our bodies are both extraordinary and intriguing.

When Jane was talking about my brain re-organising, she was talking about brain plasticity, or neuroplasticity, which I was already familiar with from having to relearn my balance after having my balance cells destroyed in my left ear to stop the horrendous, violent, vertigo of Meniere's disease.

"Neuroplasticity or brain plasticity, is defined as the ability of the nervous system to change its activity in response to intrinsic or extrinsic stimuli by reorganizing its structure, functions, or connections. A fundamental property of neurons is their ability to modify the strength and efficacy of synaptic transmission through a diverse number of activity-dependent mechanisms, typically referred as synaptic plasticity"

https://www.physio-pedia.com/Neuroplasticity
Principles of neuroplasticity

The brain wastes nothing…

So, my left hearing centre is like a baby again.

It's got me thinking.

If I was a baby again, would I choose the same path in life. For instance, if I didn't excel in sport, and I didn't receive a head trauma just in front of my left ear that I believe caused my Meniere's, would I still have Meniere's disease in my lifetime? Would I still be me?

Next: *learning to hear is like learning to read*

A Cochlear Implant is ...
addictive

Scarlett looked down for a moment then back at me. 'It's getting easier to hear with my cochlear implant, you know. And I think … I may be getting addicted to it … to hearing again.' I smiled at her words.

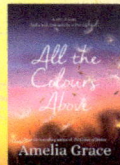

All the Colours Above
Amelia Grace

My Hearing Addiction
learning to hear is like learning to read

The rain is falling on our tin roof. I step off the veranda with my umbrella and close my eyes. A tear slips down my cheek. I can hear droplets of water battering the umbrella with two ears. For the first time in 15 years. It's a big deal. I never thought I would hear the world around me again in my left ear, except for the five torturing sounds of loud, relentless tinnitus – louder than any rock concert or loud party I had attended – a symptom of the abhorrent Meniere's disease.

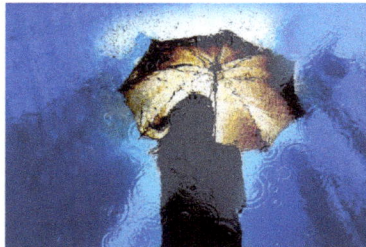

The rain is in "surround sound". It's surreal. I twirl, slowly, without losing my balance. My own type of rain dance, keeping my cochlear implant processor dry.

Bliss. *Happiness.* Beyond thankful.

My homeland, Australia, has gone from heartbreaking drought to catastrophic fires to flooding rain. But nobody is complaining. Rain is water. And water is life.

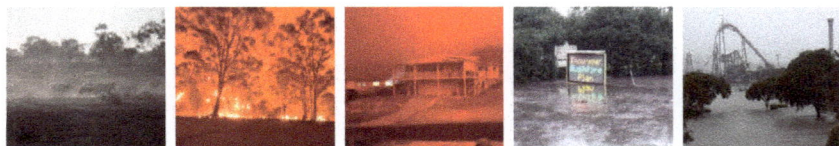

After a long moment of mindfulness, I return to my study. I have work to do. Learning to hear again. Not just sounds, but words and sentences to understand conversations to allow me to be confident with interactions with people, friends and family, and to restore my social life.

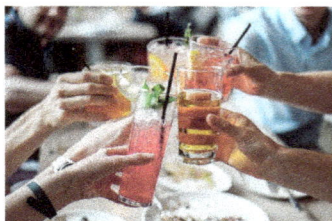

I can't lie. I was more nervous about the "switch-on" of my cochlear implant – where you finally discover if the electrodes work, how many work, and whether you can hear, or not – than the almost two-hour surgery.

I was never really certain about what I would actually hear with my cochlear implant. And there were no guarantees that I would hear well, or at all, after 15 years of deafness from Meniere's disease.

I wondered, if I could hear, would it sound like "normal"

hearing? Would I be able to understand speech? Would I be able to hear music? Or, would I be lost in a world of robotic hearing that is so terrible and irritating that I will regret having the procedure done? What *if* it is not successful? What then?

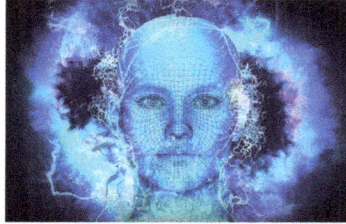

I'm taking an enormous leap of faith. I'm diving into an unknown world. How many times have I read the words,

"I'm too scared to get a cochlear implant!"

On the flip side, how many times have I read the words,

"It will change your life!"

Before being activated, I watched online cochlear implant simulators that claim to sound like what is heard with a cochlear implant, but many of them didn't sound like my implant. Mine was much better. And many were dated a very long time ago, when the technology was just new, which is old now. Hearing with a cochlear implant has come a long way since then. Cochlear implant technology has been improved and refined, so much so that surgeons are now able to apply hearing cell growth stimulator solution (gene therapy) into the cochlear with the electrodes at the time of the cochlear implant surgery. The hearing cells are stimulated to grow and attach to the electrodes to improve cochlear implant hearing even further.

Learning to hear. It's a new territory for me. A new journey. But one I am excited about.

I did a silent dance of victory when my cochlear audiologist told me I had to listen to audiobooks for at least 30 minutes a day to learn to hear. I LOVE reading!

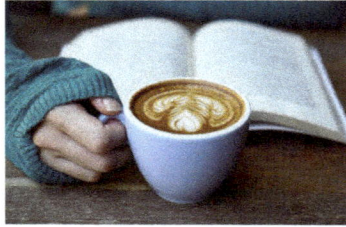

And then there were the apps for my iPhone (thanks to Apple for the direct connectivity to my CI – the *Nucleus Smart*). Apps filled with common environmental sounds; sight words; matching the sound to the visual word; matching the picture to the sound; word discrimination; sentences; and more (there's a list of apps at the end of this chapter).

The moment I started to listen to the audiobook, *The Lake House*, by Kate Morton, and followed the words in my print book, I startled.

Learning to hear is just like learning to read.

I should know. Over my teaching career, I've given thousands of students the *gift* of reading.

But with learning to hear, instead of learning what a word looks like in print, you are learning what a word sounds like. I've decided to call it a '*SoundPrint*'. I don't know whether that's a real thing, but I like the concept of it. I like the thought of making a *SoundPrint* in my cochlear implant ear to make new hearing memories, and connecting stored memories of my *once upon a time* hearing to my new hearing. It's like bringing beautiful colours of hearing back to the greyness of my deaf ear.

I've got to admit, I'm *addicted* to my cochlear implant hearing. When I don't have my CI processor on, I feel like a piece of me is missing, and I recede to my former self, the other me, all my senses on high alert. I didn't realise how exhausting my life was before my new bionic hearing.

The *gift of hearing*.

Thank you can never be enough to *Professor Graeme Clark AC*, the inventor of the multi-channel cochlear implant. My heart smiles everyday, thanks to him.

Some tips and apps I use for learning to hear:
• Join your local library so you can download audiobooks. I choose the audiobook for print books I already have at home so I can follow the printed text while listening.
• Children's picture books are highly recommended – use Storyline Online https://www.storylineonline.net/
• Cochlear CoPilot
• Hearoes
  https://www.games4hearoes.com/ FREE
• Angelsound
  http://angelsound.tigerspeech.com/ FREE
• Bring Back the Beat
• Hear Coach
• There's many more you can find with an online search. Your particular cochlear implant brand will have learning to hear apps to help your learn to hear.
• I started compiling my *Spotify* Cochlear Music Collection. But I have discovered, that if I already know the song, it is easier to understand the music with my cochlear implant hearing combined with my music memories before hearing loss.

At the end of the book, I have compiled a more detailed list.

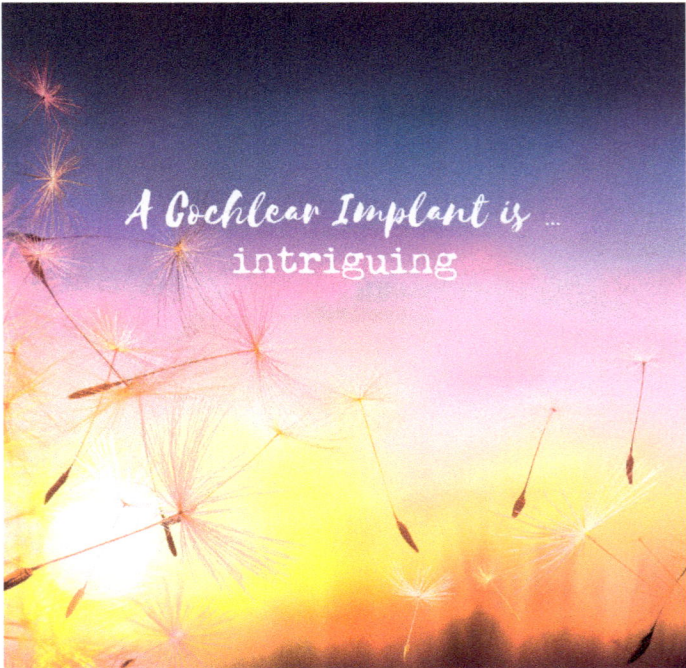

A Cochlear Implant is ...
intriguing

Friday Evening, March 20, 2020
returned natural hearing?

The cochlear implant processor rechargeable battery went flat after 13 hours of wearing my N7. That's an exceptional amount of battery time I have been told by my cochlear audiologist. I removed my processor from my head and continued writing my next novel for a little longer, saved it, then picked up my processor and carried it in my hand upstairs. I stopped at my daughter's doorway and spoke to her, casually brushing hair away from my CI ear, accidentally touching my ear, and stopped and thought, 'I can hear that.'

I fell into bed exhausted after a long day of teaching Visual Art and Music. A long day of hearing with my new cyborg ear in the classroom setting, my brain working hard to blend the two inputs of my left cochlear implant hearing and my right, good hearing ear together. Mental tiredness.

Exhaustion. An understatement … but I am glad. It means that I am making progress in relearning to hear again. Without my cochlear implant processor, I am reminded that I am deaf in my left ear by the absence of sound and awareness of my left side. The return of the dreaded loud tinnitus. I have returned to the world of one-sided hearing.

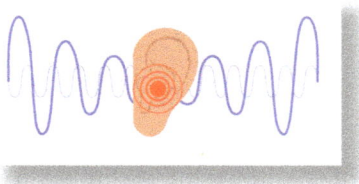

I sigh. Friyay! Yay! The weekend is here.

I roll on to my side and push my curly hair off my face, accidentally brushing over my left ear again. My cochlear implant ear. The sound of it makes me still and hold my breath. I frown.

I shouldn't be able to hear my fingers brush over my ear, the sound like rubbing your fingers over your skin, like I can hear with my good hearing ear.

That's odd.

I lift my hand to my left ear lobe again and do my scratch test. *My* scratch test. A self-learned test I have been doing for 24 years with my Meniere's disease ear to see how much I could hear on any particular day. Meniere's disease. Fluctuating hearing, one of the symptoms, until it doesn't fluctuate anymore. No hearing.

If you talk to people who have Meniere's disease, you will find that they have their own type of hearing test to determine how much they can hear on a particular day. Even Huey Lewis has his own hearing test, scratching the pillow/bed sheet to see what he could hear each morning. Then he gives it a rating out of 10.

And then there's the EarPod test. *My* EarPod test. A test I have regularly conducted in the 10 years before my cochlear implant, with hope that I had some hearing remaining, that I could still hear something. I would place the left EarPod in my Meniere's ear and stop the sound coming from the right EarPod then turn up to volume. Full Volume. The best I could hear at times was a short sharp SSH! Otherwise there was nothing. Just the sound of my disappointment.

Scratch, scratch. There. I hear it again. I wasn't imagining it. And it's loud. Normalish, like a good hearing ear would hear. A sound I haven't heard for at least 15 years with that ear.

Curious, I roll onto my back, reach for my iPhone and my wired EarPods, and plug them into my iPhone. Placing the left EarPod into my left ear only, I choose a song on my Spotify list and listen - *Light of the Seven* by Ramin Djawadi. I can hear it a little, then wonder whether my good ear is picking up the sound from the right EarPod sitting on my stomach.

So I place my hand around the right EarPod and bring it to my right ear to see if I have managed to stop sound from coming from it. It's muted quite a bit, but not entirely. So I squeeze my hand around it tighter, but still fail to stop the entirety of the music from emitting from that EarPod. So I wrap it in part of the bedcover and place it under my armpit and squeeze it tightly against me.

Success. No sound from the right EarPod.

Let the experiment with my deaf left ear begin!

I scratch my left earlobe again to check that I am not letting myself believe that I can hear something, when in fact I can't. The power of the mind.

I can still hear the ear lobe scratch, so I turn up the volume on my iPhone and listen to the song, followed by the *Star Wars* music.

I can hear it. *Perfectly.* Like I had never lost any hearing due to Meniere's disease.

Disbelief. This can't be true. There's something wrong.

Filled with adrenaline, I choose another song, this time with a person singing – *Vertigo* by Khalid. I hear his voice easily. Even the pronunciation of his words.

My breath hitches. What is going on?

I praise God for this gift, even if it is temporary, and tears trickle from my eyes. I don't understand. This isn't normal. Did my cochlear implant surgeon add some sort of solution to my cochlear before he implanted the 24 electrodes? Are the electrodes coated in something that might have affected my hearing cells?

With my heart thumping against my chest, I listen to song after song after song, all heard like I didn't have any hearing loss. I wonder, is it bone conduction?

I know all about bone hearing conduction. I was tested prior to my cochlear implant to see whether a bone conduction hearing device (also known as a BAHA) would work by transmitting sound vibrations through the bones of the skull to the cochlear of the inner ear. It didn't work. I couldn't hear a thing in my Meniere's ear.

To be doubly sure that my good ear isn't picking up the sound, I blocked my good hearing ear with noise cancelling putty, and wrapped the right-side apple EarPod numerous times in a towel so no sound came from it. I called my daughter to confirm that there was no sound, and then with my husband to make sure it just wasn't me wishfully hoping that I could hear again in my Meniere's ear.

Again, there was the music like the Meniere's Monster had never destroyed my hearing.

After listening to music in my cochlear implant ear without the processor on for an hour and a half in a state of disbelief and wonder and thankfulness, I decided to listen to some podcasts.

I can hear the speaker, but I can't quite understand the words. My heart drops a little, and I frown, baffled by what I have discovered.

Finally, I fell into deep much needed sleep.

Upon waking on Saturday morning, I tested my Meniere's ear again. The hearing was still there.

I decided to email my cochlear implant Audiologist.

Hi Jane,

Nothing urgent. I just thought I would let you know that last night I discovered I have recovered some hearing in my CI ear. I am baffled.

This is how it unfolded:

On Friday, after 13 hours wearing my processor, the battery went flat, so I removed my processor from my head. After doing some more writing on my next novel, I picked up my processor and carried it in my hand upstairs. I stopped at my daughter's doorway and spoke to her, casually brushing hair away from my CI ear accidentally touching my ear, and stopped, thinking, 'I can hear that.'

I grabbed my phone and my ear buds and put the left bud in my left ear, being careful to silence the right bud so absolutely no sound was coming from it, and holding it away from my body, and placing it underneath the bed covers to be sure that my skull wasn't picking up the sound. I checked numerous times with my daughter that she couldn't hear anything, and she couldn't. I chose a Spotify song (classical) and discovered I could hear it, with the volume on high. Not just some notes, but many notes. I tried the 'Star Wars' music, and again could hear it well. I tried two rock songs, and could hear them, one almost as if I had no hearing loss. Then I tried a podcast. I could hear the person speaking, but had no word discrimination. In a state of shock, I tried many songs on Spotify, seeing which ones I could hear and which ones I couldn't – of which I will make a list of.

Today, Saturday, I thought I would have a listen again without my processor, and I can still hear with my Meniere's ear – it is better than hearing I had over 12 years ago. And I am not sure how long it will last due to the unpredictability of Meniere's disease and the fluctuating hearing that is part of the disease. I am not sure if it has anything to do with my Meniere's disease at all. I just thought I would let you know in case it is important somehow.

Looking forward to seeing you on the 6th of April for mapping, if Attune hasn't closed due to COVID-19.

Kind regards,
Julieann Wallace
(Dip T, B. Ed, Multi-published & Bestselling Author, Artist, Teacher, Philanthropist, Tea Ninja, Chocoholic, Paper-cut Survivor)

My cochlear audiologist replied almost immediately:

Hi Julieann,

It's possible that you still have some post-operative residual hearing in that ear- we can test it when you next come in for your 3 months Ax.

Kind regards,

Jane

I replied:

Okay. That would make sense. I can also now understand speech clearly as well, which is strange. It will be reassuring to talk to you on my next visit.
See you on the 6th of April.

But the more I thought about Jane's reply, I wasn't convinced. I didn't have any residual hearing prior to the cochlear implant.

I opened up a Word Document on my computer, blocked my right ear with the sound cancelling putty, found some broken one-side working only EarPods my kids had given me (they have a weird sense of humour), and systematically went through the list of songs and music on my Spotify playlist.

This is the music I could hear perfectly, adding annotations if I couldn't hear something and what part of it was more of a challenge, or missing.

Music Only:
Handel's Water Music
Cello suite No 1 in G minor - cello
Canon in D - strings
The Swan - strings
Le reve d'lune note – piano
The Departure – Max Richter
Lovely – TwoPlusFour
Unaccompanied Cello
Hello – Henry Smith – piano
Waterfalls – Alexis French
Sail – Vitamin String Quartet
The Walker – Vitamin String Quartet
Chandelier – Vitamin String Quartet
Most music by the Vitamin String Quartet
Hurt – 2 cellos
Tetrishead – Zoe Keating - cello
One – Apocalyptica - cello
On a Cloud – Riopy – piano

Music with vocals:
Vertigo – Khalid
Closer – Skylar Grey
It's happening again – Agnes Obel

I Found – Amber Run
No Harm – Editors
Golden Brown – The Stranglers
Broken Wings – Mr. Mister
Oh Yeah – Yello – this has got a base voice – so I'm surprised
I can hear this song.
Do You Remember – Jarryd James
Trauma – NF
Marathon – Gem Club
Sorry – Aquilo
Trampoline – Shaed
Until We Go Down – Ruelle
Contaminated – Banks
Born in a Slumber – Flora Cash
Oblivion – Labrinth
Gameshow – Two Door Cinema Club
Lavendar – Two Door Cinema Club
Gasoline – Two Door Cinema Club
You Love Me – Flora Cash
Silhouette – Aquilo
Wildfire – SYML
Mr. Sandman – SYML
I Speak Jesus – Here be Lions, Darlene Zschech
Good Good Father – Chris Tomlin
Anything with piano
Anything with strings
Dance Monkey – Tone And I
Never Seen the Rain – Tone And I
Waymaker – Michael W. Smith
Tremble – Nicole Miller

I kept listening to music going down the list of my playlist, but stopped writing down the tiles and artists, as I could hear them all. Well.

Then I decided to listen to PODCASTS again, adding notes about what I could hear.

Podcasts

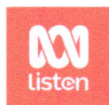

ABC News

Should you just pull your kid out of school? Dr Norman Swan – I can understand his speech. Today it sounds like normal speech.

California Goes into Lockdown – Sabra Lane – I can hear her pronunciation perfectly.

Covid – 19 Lessons from Singapore and Taiwan – Geralkdine Doogue

Why is it so cold in here? – Robyn Williams – I can understand words but a little harder to work out some words.

I can hear men's voices

Stop Everything – Benjamin Law and Beverley Wang – understood perfectly.

Ted talks

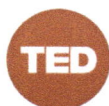

Go ahead, dream about the future – understood easily

How You can support farmers in the US – Eric Sannerud - understood easily

What investigating neural pathways can reveal about mental

health – Kay M. Tye – easy

How Technology has changed what it's like to be deaf – Rebecca Krill – easy

The beautiful, hard work of co-parenting – Joel Leon – easy

Why books are here to stay – Chip Kidd – understand most

How the compass unlocked the world – David Biello – easy

Epic engineering: building the Brooklyn Bridge – Alex Gendler - easy

How to know it's time to change careers – Chieh Huang - easy

I stopped and removed the EarPod. I'm quite certain I have proven the point that I can hear in my Meniere's ear without my processor on, with the volume on high. Three weeks until my next cochlear implant mapping appointment. Maybe I will find answers then?

A Cochlear Implant is ...
a commitment

The more you use it,
the easier and better it gets.

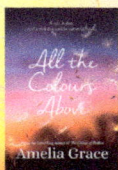

Monday April 6, 2020
3 month cochlear implant mapping

It's an eerie drive to the city for my 3 month cochlear implant mapping session today. COVID. The city is like a ghost town. We've just come out of a strict lock-down. Except for me. I am classified as an essential worker as a teacher, and still had to go to school. We had just spent a week making critical changes to teaching plans to deliver lessons to students online and in class. A change to teaching that would be happening after the two week school holiday break.

But for today, I was keen for this appointment to have a hearing test as well as my cochlear implant mapping.

The reception area to the audiologists' rooms is empty. The endless magazines that adorned the table in the middle of the room was bare.

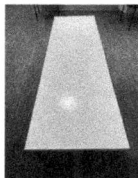

All magazines, books and charts had been removed so that no personalisation was left. Anything that could be handled by people was gone.

I was by myself today. My husband who came to every appointment was not allowed to attend due to COVID. He waited for me downstairs in the foyer of the building.

Jane entered the reception area and quickly lead me to her room for mapping, for fine tuning my cochlear implant again.

There was no smile, the universal body language for welcome. Everything was done with speed and a sense of urgency in her voice. The unknowns of COVID in 2020 had everyone on edge.

She quickly connected my N7 to her computer and tapped a few keys to download the data from my cochlear implant, and then conducted the mapping of my cochlear implant. It wasn't a full mapping, just a brief one, where she adjusted a couple of electrodes so I could hear better.

Again, this mapping did not fail to impress me with the entire technology of cochlear implant hearing. It's mind-blowing.

'Can you please explain to me why I can hear almost perfectly in my Meniere's ear?' I asked with curiosity. I needed answers for being able to miraculously hear out of my deaf ear again.

Jane took a deep breath then turned towards me. 'It can only be residual hearing that was preserved when your surgeon performed the procedure.'

I shook my head. 'But I didn't have any hearing before the procedure.'

'You'll have to talk to your surgeon about it.'

I nodded. I would be seeing him in three months time. 'Can you please give me a hearing test for my natural hearing in my left ear. I need to know whether what I was hearing at home is true.'

Jane blinked after a moment in time. I could see that she didn't really want to do a hearing test on my left ear. 'I'll give you a quick hearing test. Let's go.'

Relieved I stood, then watched her disinfect everywhere I had touched, including my seat. My stomach gave a nervous quiver. This COVID stuff was real.

I followed her with quick steps to a sound proof hearing test room. Before she attached the necessary equipment for the hearing test, she disinfected it.

'We're on limited time. This will be a short.'

I nodded, ecstatic to be doing a hearing test.

Jane put the ear muffs over my ears, gave me a button to push, added loud background grey noise into my right ear, then proceeded to do the word discrimination test in my left ear.

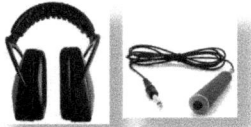

I struggled to hear words clearly. But I could hear better than before, which was nothing. This time I could hear the "shape" of words. I haven't heard that in about 15 years. Something has definitely changed.

After only four attempts at repeating words, Jane stops the hearing test and removes the push button from me, disinfecting it, then the ear muffs, disinfecting them, and asks me to stand.

'Your hearing is still the same,' she says, then methodically disinfects the seat and also where she has used the audiology technology.

Before I can try to explain to her what I can hear, we swiftly leave the room and she leads me to the reception desk where I book my next mapping session for the six month checkup, standing behind a yellow line masked onto the floor to stop the spread of any airborne virus droplets.

This is the most rushed mapping and hearing appointment I have ever had. I am going to return home without answers I was looking for. But I'm not angry with Jane. I'm not unhappy with the mapping session. She has fine tuned my hearing so it is clearer and I have improved my word recognition test. COVID is the problem. It has infected everyone with fear.

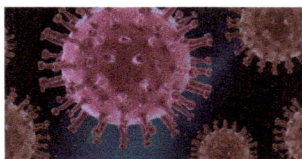

July, 2020
6 month cochlear implant mapping & cochlear implant surgeon

The reception area of the audiologist has changed again. There are far fewer chairs. The ones remaining as spaced apart like we are being disciplined by the head master.

The absence of magazines on the table and the request to wear masks reminds me that we are not out of the COVID danger yet.

'Julieann.' I hear her clearly. I look up to see Jane. My cochlear implant has blended the sounds from both ears and she sounds normal. She has a blue mask on covering her mouth and nose, but I think I can see her eyes smiling at me. I stand and follow her to her room.

The six month mapping session is longer this time compared to the rushed COVID April appointment. It's thorough, starting with connecting my processor to the computer and checking the data, like how many electrodes are working, how long I wear the processor for each day, the battery life each day, how much time

I spend listening to speech, and to music. Jane blocks the hearing in my good ear then fine tunes my cochlear implant hearing using the beeping sounds. My hearing is even better.

'Can you hear this?' she rattles a piece of paper in front of her.

'Yes,' I say, although it doesn't sound like paper, but an unrecognisable noise.

She stands and goes behind me and rubs a tissue to see if I can hear it. I nod. She rattles some paper that I can hear. She asks me to repeat words that she says, her mask covering her mouth so I can't lip read. I understand 99%.

I listen to sentences and repeat them back. Jane is impressed. She goes to another room and says words and letter blends I need to repeat for her. I get 80% correct. Jane is thrilled by my progress, considering I was deaf in my Meniere's ear for 15 years, and there were no guarantees of how well I would hear again.

All fine tuned with my mapping and ready to go, I book my one year mapping session for January 2021, then catch the elevator down a couple of floors for my ENT surgeon appointment.

'Julieann.' My ENT surgeon's voice is easy to hear. I look up, stand, and follow him to his room. He speaks with a mask over his nose and mouth for COVID protection, but I easily understand every word that is spoken.

'Is it okay to speak to you with my mask on?' he asks.

'Yes. I understand every word you are saying,' I answer.

'Good. How are you and how is your implant going?' he asks.

'I'm well and my CI is amazing, thanks to you,' I say.

He nods. He has already seen the results of my mapping sessions from my cochlear audiologist, Jane, and comments on how well I am doing with my hearing progress, then removes my processor, checks the scar behind my left ear to see how it is healing, and then the position of the cochlear implant under my skin. He is pleased.

He looks inside ear of my ear canals, and removes some ear wax from my good ear.

'I can hear in my deaf ear again really well without the processor on,' I say.

His expression doesn't change.

'Did you add anything inside my cochlear when you did the surgery?'

He shakes his head then says, 'I don't have an explanation for what you can hear again.'

I am shocked by how he brushes off my question. But I'm also aware that we are on a tight time schedule due to COVID.

I'm disappointed, but I understand.

A Cochlear Implant ...
changed my life

- I forget that I am deaf in my left ear. It **IS** that good!
- I feel balanced. A feeling of freedom.
- Listening to music with my CI ear and my good ear gives me a natural addictive high - it's called a binaural beat.
- I am happier.
- I can hear better than other hearing people in noisy social settings at times.
- I don't have to keep asking people to repeat themselves.
- People have no idea I have hearing loss.
- When I am wearing my processor, I feel safe when out and about.
- I have no tinnitus when wearing my processor.

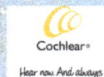

Cochlear®

Hear now. And always

Julieann Wallace ~ author, artist, teacher, philanthropist, paper cut survivor

Meniere's disease is ...
frustrating

It's my life, my illness ...
Please let me
choose my treatment

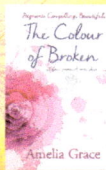

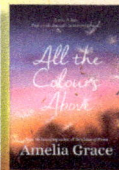

It's My Life, My Illness …
please let me choose my treatment

'I'm sorry. There is no cure.'

I *die a little inside* each time I hear someone with Meniere's disease pleading for help, saying they can't do it anymore, and when I hear the call-out for prayer for someone who is suicidal from the insidious incurable Meniere's disease … I've been there. I know exactly how it feels.

I wish I had a magic wand to heal every one of us. Right now.

I get angry when I read Meniere's patients being told by their doctors, 'I'm sorry. There is nothing more we can do.'

Don't accept it. There is more that can be done.

But … it also depends on what *you are willing to do*.

Let me tell you the short story version of my journey.

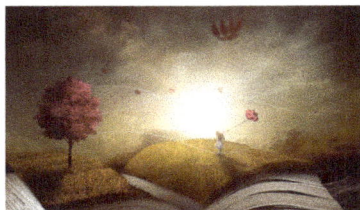

1995 …

'I'm sorry. There is no cure.'

'No cure?'

'No … no cure. No cause. But you're not going to die from it.' My ear specialist eyed me with caution. The bitterness of my diagnosis after five hours of testing was painful to acknowledge.

'Let's wait and see how your symptoms go,' he said.

I stepped out of the ENT's office, trailed by a very dark shadow: Meniere's disease. It was so large it cast a darkness over me like a heavy storm cloud, ready to erupt into the strong spiralling wind of a cyclone at any moment.

I knew the symptoms of my diagnosis well.

I lived them with every breath that I took, mixed with fear and anxiety: aural fullness, hearing loss, tinnitus, and vertigo – *the abhorrent violent vertigo* – a life destroyer.

I felt like I was given a prison sentence.

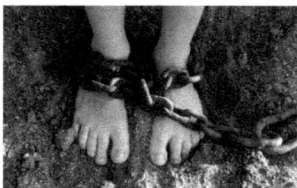

Where was the key to escape from Meniere's disease?

Wait and see how my symptoms go?

Why?

'You could have a mild form of Meniere's disease that has little impact on your life, or it could go into remission,' he had said.

But mine didn't.

Symptoms of Meniere's Disease

- Hearing loss
- Spontaneous, violent vertigo
- Nausea
- Vomiting
- Ear fullness and sometimes pain
- Tinnitus
- Hearing loss
- Deafness
- Nystagmus
- Extreme fatigue
- Mental disorientation at times
- Imbalance
- Mood swings
- Hyperacusis
- Anxiety
- Depression

After return visits to my ENT I was given a diuretic and Stemetil. That was it. And that was all they had in 1996.

End of story.

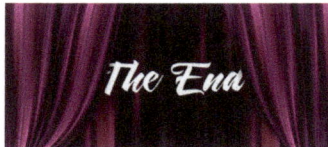

The End

But was it?

As my Meniere's disease kicked into overdrive, destroying every bit of happiness I had in my life, the worst my ENT had seen, I got up to fight. Life was brutally unfair. Why was Meniere's disease even a thing? It's so cruel.

I was angry. I wasn't going to accept "there's no more we can do".

So I took control.

1. I started journaling my lifestyle - vertigo attacks, what I did, ate, or drank before an episode, trying to find a trigger or a pattern – and I discovered one – every two months I would have four hours of violent vertigo for nine days in a fortnight. Sometimes ending up in hospital.

2. I started my own research online when we finally had a home computer.

3. I researched and tried natural therapies.

4. I tried acupuncture.

5. I had my jaw alignment checked for TMJ (temporomandibular joint).

6. I listened to sound therapy for months on end – the Tomatis effect.

7. I took my research to my ENT, every visit. I'm sure he let out a sigh every time he saw my name on his patient list for the day. And when I found a Japanese doctor who claimed that the anti-viral Acyclovir cured people of their Meniere's disease, my ENT was doubtful, but told me to give it a go. It cost me around $375 for each script from my GP – and that's another story. It didn't work.

8. I tried Serc in 2002.

But still, the debilitating vertigo rendered me defenseless. Incapacitated. And mentally, I found myself at the bottom of the darkest abyss with no hope, wearing a mask with a smile, covering up my very, very deep and dark depression.

2004 ...

1. I tried prednisone. For one day I felt like a normal person. And then my vertigo returned.

2. I had a grommet inserted into my eardrum. It did nothing.

The doctor's words were full of apology. And frustration. 'I'm sorry. There is nothing more we can do.'

'Nothing more?' My heart dropped. There was no horizon of hope like the sun's rays projecting onto the twilight canvas. It had disappeared into the darkness. Like me.

Just me and the beast: Meniere's.

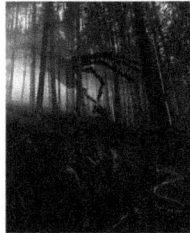

My ENT looked gutted. 'Well ... we could try gentamicin injected into your middle ear, and if that doesn't work, I can do a vestibular nerve section.'

'I'll take the gentamicin.'

'It will destroy your balance cells. You will also lose some hearing.'

'Does it stop the vertigo?'

'It can. Yes.'

'Then I'll take the gentamicin.' I didn't care about losing more hearing. I couldn't live with the vertigo.

I was done …

From years of experience, I *know* that more can be done.

There is more that can be done ...
depending on ...

1. *Have you got the correct diagnosis?*
What if you don't have Meniere's disease, but have an ailment, that when diagnosed correctly, is easily fixed?

2. *Your ENT*
Do they understand and listen to what's happening to you, not only physically, but psychologically, socially, emotionally - how is your mental health? Are they supportive of your requests and treatment options?

3. *What are **you** willing to do?*
My ENT working through the list of least invasive treatments to invasive. I couldn't do the violent vertigo attacks anymore. I was done. My Ent said I was the worst MD patient he had seen. When, or if you are given options by your ENT, work through the pros and cons of each treatment to see if it is right for you.

2020 …

I've been vertigo free since 2004. But the gentamicin injected into my middle ear was not the low dose gentamicin offered now, it was the full strength, and I remember my ENT saying that he added bi-carbonate of soda and sterile water to the mix to make the toxic antibiotic penetrate better. I now have my life back. And my shadow, Meniere's, is a small thing that follows me around, a reminder that I am a survivor and a fighter.

I have to admit, I'm a little jealous of newly diagnosed Meniere's people now. You have so much more HOPE than I did when I started my Meniere's journey in 1995. There are far more medications and treatment options and success stories, and support groups and people who have started blogs and websites and Zoom sessions for MD people.

You *have* so much more.

And remember, you *can* choose. Like I did. Make sure you have a supportive ENT. I'm eternally thankful to my ENT and his care and compassion. And now my new ENT for his skill with my cochlear implant that has allowed me to hear again after 15 years.

Meniere's Warriors …

It's your life.

Be proactive.

Take control.

This is your weapon -

Research

Scour the Internet for everything about Meniere's disease and treatment options. Present them to your ENT. You are your best advocate. It's your life. You take control.

This is your plan -

Trial

Trial approaches and treatments that people are having successes with (after researching – there's a lot of scammers/snake oil salespeople/quacks out there trying to make money out of our suffering).

This is your mantra -

Never give up!

Reach out. Join groups. Meet others with Meniere's disease in person. We've got this, together.

This is your to do -

Keep a journal

Make your own journal or buy one, or perhaps there's an App you can download. Keep a list of activities, food, drink, stresses, weather, headaches/migraines, jaw alignment, neck pain etc. It may help you to find a pattern or trigger.

3 Month Daily Meniere's Journal created by me. All profits are donated to Meniere's research. Available at online bookstores.

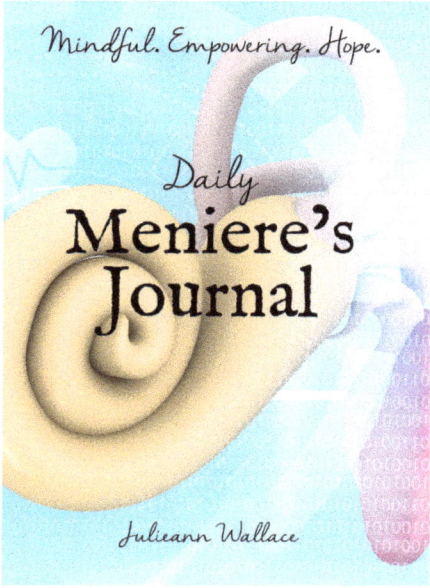

Mindful. Empowering. Hope.

Daily
**Meniere's
Journal**

Julieann Wallace

About the
Daily Meniere's Journal

My shadow, Meniere's, has been with me for 26 years at the time of this journal publication. A very difficult 26 years, where in the first 10 years, I would be debilitated for 4 hours or more at a time with horrendous violent vertigo. Meniere's an absolute life changer. I developed a chronic fear of vertigo attacks, and PTSD, and so stopped shopping, socialising, driving, and teaching. Everyday I kept a diary of what I ate or drank, where I had been and what I had done, to see if I could find the trigger for my attacks.

It is my hope that this journal can help you. Each page has a table of *Symptoms*, and of *What Helped Me!* Add information to *Weather, Food* and *Other Triggers*. By keeping a track of your daily living with Meniere's, you may find a pattern that will help you with your battle against it. As you are using the journal, highlight symptoms you have on that day, add notes about what you are experiencing, or any new symptoms, plus vertigo length and severity. Please be aware that I have added BPPV* (Benign Paroxysmal Positional Vertigo - a problem with the crystals in the inner ear - symptoms are brief periods of vertigo, that is, of a spinning sensation upon changes in the position of the head, lasting less than a minute). BPPV is NOT a symptom of Meniere's. You can have Meniere's and BPPV at the same time. BPPV has a technique called the *Epley Manoeuvre* that can stop those episodes.

Because this is your journal, you can add your own stamp and style. Glue in prayers, inspirational verses or images that speak to you in some way. Be creative, be arty. I have added pages of light text at the end of each month, where you can draw or paint artwork over the top, or glue notes you have written, or letters to yourself etc. Being a Secondary Art Teacher, I know the value of art as a tool for healing and restoration when words are simply not enough.

Three Things I am Thankful For Today - When I was struggling in a deep and dark depression with my Meniere's in the early 2000's, I learned the value of finding things I was thankful for. Everyday. Single. Day. No matter how small. This act of focusing is now called 'Mindfulness', and is very powerful. As you travel daily with your Meniere's, remember, **you are a warrior. You've got this!**

It is my forever hope and prayer, that a cure is found.

Julieann xo

MONTH: January February March April May June July
August September October November December

Day: Monday Tuesday Wednesday Thursday Friday Saturday Sunday
Date: _____ Season: Summer Autumn/Fall Winter Spring
Temperature: Low _____ High _____
Barometer: 9am _____ 9pm _____ Humidity _____

Sunny	Cloudy	Rain	Showers	Windy
Snow	Storm	Humid	Dry	

Food & Fluid Intake (be mindful of salt):

Breakfast			
Lunch			
Dinner			
Fluid Intake	Water -		
Snacks			

Symptoms:

Tinnitus	Vertigo	Drop Attack	Nausea
Anxiety	Brain Fog	Hearing Loss	Hyperacusis
Fatigue	Balance	Co-ordination	Stress
Headache	Migraine	Nystagmus	Disequilibrium
Ear Fullness/ Pressure/Pain	Vision Difficulties	Physical Impairment	Vestibular Migraine
Vomiting	Depression	BPPV*	Diarrhea
PPPD*	Jaw Click/Pain	Neck Pain	Motion Sensitivity
Sweating	Speech Difficulty	Monthly Cycle	

29

What time did your symptoms start?
Tinnitus: L R How many noises? _____ Loudness Scale: 1 2 3 4 5
Possible Meniere's Symptom Triggers Today:
Physical: _____

_____ Pollen, Mold, Dust, Trees, Grass, Ragweed
Visual: _____

Emotional: _____

What Helped Me?

Medication/s & Time Taken	Other	
	Prayer	Rest
	Meditation	Friend/s
	Self-care	Family
	Exercise	Pet/s
	Mindfulness	Vestibular Rehab
	Gratitude	Hearing Device

Duration of Vertigo _____ minutes _____ hours _____ days
Severity of Vertigo 1 2 3 4 5 - I HATE you, vertigo!
New Symptoms? _____

What I Accomplished Today – Something to Celebrate!

Three Things I am Thankful for Today:
1.
2.
3.

Meniere's Survival Mode

- *Seek* medical help
- *Educate* yourself so you are a Meniere's Ninja!
- *Join* support groups online and in person
- *Know that you will experience grief* (not necessarily in the order, and not necessarily all of them)
  Denial
  Anger
  Bargaining
  Depression
  Acceptance
- You may experience anxiety and/or depression - *educate* yourself about it and *seek help* (cognitive behaviour therapy or medical help or medicine). You don't need to suffer through these.

Meniere's Super Survival Mode

- *Find 3 things you are thankful for.* Every. Single. Day.
- *Do something you can achieve* - even if it is just getting out of bed in the morning.
- *Do something that you love* - no matter how insignificant others think it is.
- *Distract yourself.*
- *Don't put off any treatments* - don't wait e.g. medications, hearing devices etc

Doctors, this is our plea: *please let us choose our steps to wellness, to a better life where we can find joy again, where we can take back what Meniere's disease has taken from us. Please don't say "there is nothing more you can do".* We have suffered more than enough.

The same applies to hearing loss:

Doctors, this is our plea: *please let us choose our steps to hearing again, to a better life where we can find joy again, where we can take back what hearing loss has taken from us. Please don't say "there is nothing more you can do".* We know there is more.

A Cochlear Implant is ...
cutting edge technology

'How's your cochlear implant?' Tobi said.
'Great. Amazing!' Scarlett said.
'I've heard the technology is quite advanced now,' he said.
'It is.'

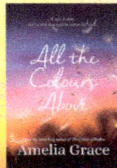

January, 2021
one year mapping appointment

Summer = Heat + Humidity, in Queensland, Australia, and with it comes the seasonal quest of trying to stay cool, somehow, hating that dreaded humidity that makes your skin sticky like you need to take a hundred showers a day. And when you do step out the shower, you start sweating all over again. My shadow, Meniere's, raises his hand then takes a bow, loving this hot weather and the rain that comes with it, the low pressure systems affecting my tinnitus and my balance, leaving me with nausea. Crystalised ginger is my go to. It stops the nausea better than Stemetil. Summer is my least favourite season in living with Meniere's.

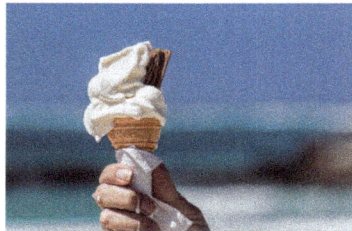

I wipe the perspiration beads from my forehead, glad to be getting in the air-conditioned car. A short reprieve while my husband drives to the city for 45 minutes.

The heat knocks me when I get out of the car to make my escape into the air-conditioned building. Another reprieve.

3rd floor. No magazines on the coffee table. Chairs are spaced out like we have been put into timeout. COVID is still making its presence felt.

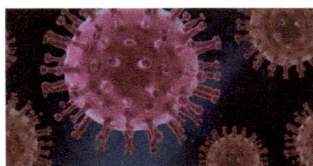

Jane doesn't greet me with a smile. She's on holidays. Instead I have Josh. I can't tell if he greets me with a smile because he has a mask on. My shadow, Meniere's, and I follow him to Jane's office. My unfriends, Anxiety, Tinnitus and Deafness don't accompany me. None of them exist at this visit because of my cochlear implant.

Josh attaches my processor to the computer and looks at the collected data. He fines tunes my mapping a little more, then tests my word discrimination. 99%. He looks back at my records and discovers I had 0% word discrimination before my CI. He's impressed. And so am I.

'You've worked well to get your results. There's people who get a cochlear implant but don't come to mapping appointments. They are the ones who don't make much progress.'

I am surprised. I wonder why you would bother to get a cochlear implant if you weren't going to put 100% effort into relearning to hear again. Their loss I guess. This technology is a life changer.

'I'm interested in the off the ear processor,' I tell Josh. 'When I take off my COVID mask I tend to knock off my processor when the mask elastic catches on my over-the-ear component. The US already has the Kanso 2. When will it be here in Australia, where they invented it?'

'It's coming this year. I'll let Jane know that you are interested in one.'

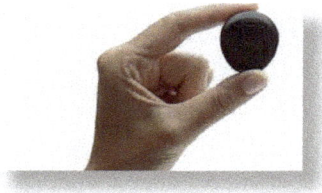

July, 2021

It's a cold winter's day outside - 20°C maximum (I know, 20°C, I can hear you laughing if you live in a country where it snows). I'm sitting in a room of people eager to learn about the Kanso 2 and to try one on their head. I'm the youngest person here by about 20 years. I glance out the window and gaze at the beautiful blue sky like a dome over us. It reminds me of the miracle of the earth and our oxygen supply. I return my focus back to the representative from Cochlear Australia talking about the off the ear Kanso 2. All of the elderly cochlear implant N7 wearers, like me, are nodding their heads, but I am smiling. An off the ear processor would be amazing.

To my surprise, we are all handed a Kanso 2 that has been pre-loaded with our hearing map ready to try on. I remove my N7 processor and attach the Kanso 2 to my head. It's so light. It's comfortable. I talk to my husband. I watch the other CI people, some liking it, some not, some undecided. My mind wanders for a moment, wondering about their cochlear implant journey. How did they lose their hearing?

I need to test something out with the Kanso 2, and so I stand, then jump up and down. I'm the only one in the room who does this. I see my cochlear implant audiologist, Jane, and the Cochlear Australia presenter smile at me. I want to know if the device will fall off my head with movement like that.

It stays put. It has passed my test and I am impressed!

I put my order in for a Kanso 2. It arrives in August two days before my birthday and I return to the city for Jane to fit it, check the mapping and explain how to care for it.

I leave her office filled with joy, my shadow, Meniere's, following me with crossed arms and a grumpy look on his face.

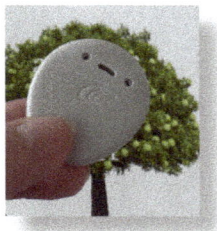

A Cochlear Implant is ...
beyond amazing

- I have direction of hearing - it makes me feel safe.
- I can direct stream music or podcasts to my cochlear implant while I am working, and no one knows.
- I tell my students at school that I can hear what they think! At first they always believe me (the look on their faces is priceless). It makes them wonder for a moment, before I let them off the hook. Luckily they have a sense of humour.
- I have an advantage of being able to use my lip and body language reading skills as well as hearing speech. A gift.

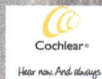

Cochlear®
Hear now. And always.

Julieann Wallace – author, artist, teacher, philanthropist, paper cut survivor

A Cochlear Implant is ...
life changing

'Thank you for encouraging me to get a
cochlear implant, it has changed my life.
I don't think I could live without it now.'
Scarlett ran her hand over her facial tattoo.

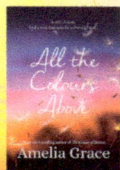

January, 2022
two year mapping appointment

I look up when I hear my name called.

Jane, my cochlear audiologist greets me with a smile. The universal language that puts you at ease, *perhaps*. I can't tell because of the COVID mask she is wearing. Instead, I judge by the sound of her voice. My Shadow, Meniere's, my husband, and I follow her to her office. We all sit down, except for my shadow, Meniere's. He's sitting in the corner, sulking. He doesn't like losing at the game of Meniere's. I have eliminated the vertigo with gentamicin, had balance rehabilitation and have returned my hearing with the help of technology, which also stops the tinnitus when I am wearing the cochlear implant processor.

'Welcome back,' Jane says through her mask. 'Would you like me to remove my mask so you can understand me better?'

'No,' I say. 'I can understand you perfectly with your mask on. I've had lots of practise at hearing without reading lips because of the masks.'

Her eyes crinkle. She's smiling.

Jane hooks me up to the computer to read my data that is recorded in my processor. She checks how many hours a day I wear my processor. She checks how many hours I am engaged in listening to speech and music.

'You are doing well with your cochlear implant,' she says. 'We didn't expect you to do so well considering you were deaf in your Meniere's ear for fifteen years beforehand.' She shakes her head. 'It's amazing!'

Jane checks the cochlear implant mapping, then plays sounds on it to check my hearing. She only adjusts one of the electrodes.

'I've seen other cochlear implant wearers with bass and treble adjustments enabled on their Nucleus Smart App. I'd like that as well,' I say.

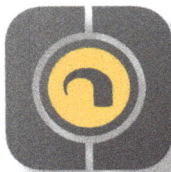

Jane taps a few keys on her computer and explains the feature to me. 'You have already had the sensitivity setting added. I have now added bass control and treble control. You can adjust these to suit the environment you are in. I'll also re-add the music setting.'

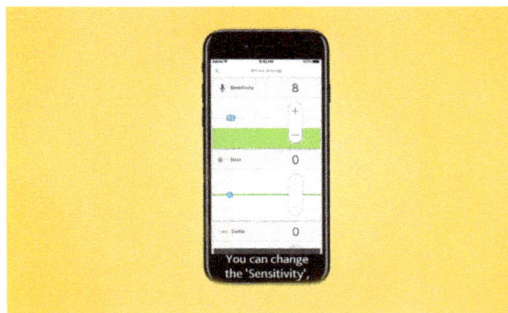

I think back to my last mapping a year ago. Josh asked me whether I used the music setting on my cochlear implant and I said not much. So he removed it with my permission.

'Thanks,' I say. 'I prefer to have the choice of using the music setting if I want. It gives me more control over my listening experience.'

Jane uses a foam ear plug in my good ear, then places ear phones over my good ear as well. It stops all sound from entering my good ear. She tests my cochlear implant hearing by interacting with speech with me, then goes into a sound proof room behind me and asks me to repeat what I hear.

She returns to the room. 'Excellent. 99% word discrimination.'

I smile. I know that my cyborg hearing is amazing, but the numerous tests I do with her confirm that I am able to hear so well.

I am so thankful for this technology.

Jane leads my husband and I out of her office to the reception area. I'm dragging my shadow, Meniere's, out by the foot. He's a sore loser.

A Cochlear Implant is ...
life changing

Gram has a cochlear implant now.
It changed her life! It's like she's back to her
old self before Meniere's disease, the ugly
life-stealer! She's just so ... happy!

February, 2022
cochlear implant surgeon appointment

My shadow, Meniere's, is hanging on to my dress like a shy child. We've entered the empty ENT reception for my two year appointment with my cochlear implant surgeon. I'm the only one in the waiting room, besides my shadow, Meniere's. COVID is still impacting us, globally.

'Julieann?'

I look up to see my doctor and smile behind my COVID mask. I follow him to his room, and my shadow, Meniere's, sits under my chair, hiding from the doctor imbued with Meniere's disease knowledge, who is also my cochlear implant surgeon. Talented.

'Do you need me to remove my mask?' he asks, implying is it easier for me to understand him without his mask and also read his lips.

'No,' I say. 'I can hear you perfectly well.'

He nods, then checks my cochlear implant scar. He removes

my Kanso 2 and feels for the position of the implant under my skin above my left ear. He grabs his otoscope to check inside my ears.

'Everything looks great. Is there anything you are worried about, or any problems with your cochlear implant?'

'None. I'm just so thankful for the technology, and for you, who did such a great job with the surgery.'

His eyes smile. 'I wish everyone was like you. There are some cochlear implant recipients who complain that the cochlear implant doesn't work. They think that getting a CI is like turning on a light. Once they have "switch-on", they expect to hear perfectly again without any effort on their part.'

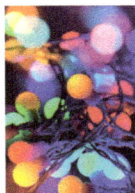

I frown. Everyone who goes through the process to see whether they are a candidate for a cochlear implant is told about how they have to work towards relearning to hear.

'I worked hard to relearn to hear. I did all the recommended exercises, plus more, even finding apps to use to enhance my cochlear implant hearing. You get out of it what you put into it,' I say.

'Exactly,' he said. He wrote down some notes on my file, then said, 'I very happy with your cochlear implant. I won't need to see you anymore, unless there is a problem.'

This was something unexpected. 'Really?'

He nodded.

I thanked my amazing surgeon, then left his room with my

shadow, Meniere's, running quick steps to keep up with me.

It hits me again that I have been freed from the symptoms of Meniere's disease. My eyes fill with tears.

What a journey.

What a victory.

So thankful.

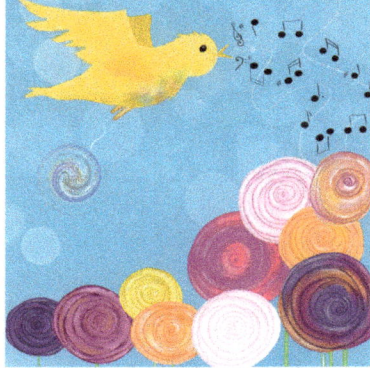

Freed. ♡

Beyond thankful. Embrace life. It's a gift. The colour of happy. Love with all my heart. Fearless. Never forget my journey.

A Cochlear Implant is ...
innovative

'And,' I signed, 'they are also trialling gene therapy with cochlear implants, where they inject a DNA solution into the cochlear before the implant, and then fire electrical impulses to trigger the DNA transfer once the implant is inserted. It will allow regrowth of auditory nerves to regain hearing.

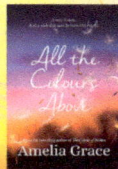

All the Colours About
Amelia Grace

Friday May 27th, 2022
invitation to macquarie university

Look for the helpers. That's always my go to when something not so good happens. The helpers, the heroes, are always somewhere out of eyesight, but when the time is needed, they appear, as if called.

My friend, Dizzy Anne, is one of those helpers. She has been instrumental in organising meet-ups, websites and Zoom meetings with information sessions for people with Meniere's disease. One day she sent out an email. It was an invitation to visit the Macquarie University in Sydney for a tour of the School of Engineering for Meniere's disease, and the Cochlear Hearing Hub.

Instead of excited at the invitation, my heart dropped. I lived in a different state of Australia and Wednesday was one of my teaching days.

I couldn't go.

After letting the disappointment settle for a couple of days, I decided to take the day off school and fly down to Sydney for the tour. I have been donating a lot of money to Meniere's disease research after all. Plus, in my latest novel, *All the Colours Above,* the Meniere's researcher cures Meniere's disease with a nanorobotics. Were they doing this now at the Meniere's research centre?

The flights were booked to Sydney and school is organised for me to be away. Can't wait to be there, and to meet Dizzy Anne for the first time in person!

Will it feel strange meeting other people with Meniere's disease, like me?

Thursday June 16th, 2022
macquarie university tour

It's early in the morning and I'm buzzing with excess energy. I'm restless, and failing at trying to focus on getting ready to go to work to teach secondary students. My thoughts are all over the place and I'm filled with an ocean of hope for the future of Meniere's disease. It's also the day *after* I flew to Sydney to attend the Macquarie University for a tour of the School of Engineering and Hearing Hub. Yes, I wagged school to fly interstate. It's for a cochlear appointment I told my employer, leaving out the fact that the appointment was a 1hr 35min flight to Sydney.

Yesterday, I was up at 4:30am to catch a flight to Sydney. After the flight I caught three trains to the Macquarie University Train Station. Anne said she would meet us here. I looked around. No Anne. Maybe she meant not right here, but at the entrance of the station. I looked up at the exit. Two massive escalators, around 100 steps each. How far underground were we?

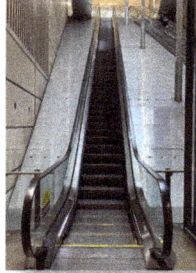

I reached the top of the station and stepped out into the bright daylight and looked up. It was such a beautiful day in Sydney.

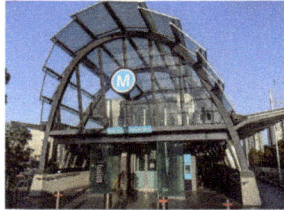

'Julieann?'

I shifted my gaze expecting to see Anne. Dizzy Anne. But it wasn't her. 'Yes,' I said, assuming it was one of the thirteen Meniere's people who were gathering at the Macquarie University today.

'I'm Eleanor. I recognise you from the Zoom sessions.'

I smiled then remembered I was a Meniere's guest speaker at one of Sydney Meniere's Group Zoom sessions. Technology connecting us globally. 'Hi, Eleanor.'

And then our conversation started. Eleanor told me her Meniere's story and I asked her questions. At once her Meniere's traits appeared, those traits that people with Meniere's know so well. That turn of the head to the better hearing ear. The "can you say that again?" request. The stop in the conversation when the traffic noise became too loud. What a terrible place to share stories. I watched once again as she turned her good ear toward me to hear what I was saying. My heart cracked. That was me once, trying to listen, trying to lip read, trying to fill in the missing or misheard words to make sense of what was being said, the nodding and smiling when I should have been answering a question. Eleanor needs a cochlear implant. Like me. It would make her life so much easier. Dear, dear Eleanor. I wanted to hug her so tightly that all her broken bits from Meniere's would be pushed back together. Her life story … I took a deep breath, what a strong woman she is. I was in awe of her.

And then Annette appeared. Annette knew my name before I could say anything. She told me her Meniere's story. It was her neck that was out, and once she had it worked on, she hadn't had vertigo since, but she still has the other symptoms.

Then Anne appeared. The shaker and mover, Dizzy Anne. The Anne who started the *Sydney Meniere's Support Group* (https://sydneymenieressupportgroup.com/). *The* Anne who organises regular and popular Zoom meetings with guest speakers to educate, support and help people with Meniere's disease - *Meniere's Support Group - Dizzy Anne - YouTube*. Legendary Anne with a heart of gold.

More people appeared as if from nowhere. A head count. Two people were missing. They couldn't make it. We all understood perfectly. That horrid beast of Meniere's disease. You can make plans, but it is the Meniere's Monster that destroys them for you.

My heart sank for them and I started to slip into that dark, dark place of long ago when that was me. When Meniere's had taken so much away from my life and I was on my hands and knees trying to find the missing pieces of me. I lifted my face to the sunshine, thankful for my Meniere's journey, thankful that I was able to be a voice for sufferers, and thankful that I was here today to meet the researchers working to find a cure for us. It must be coming soon.

Hope.

After finding our bearings we were on the move, headed toward the Macquarie University Hearing Hub Café where our day of insight would begin.

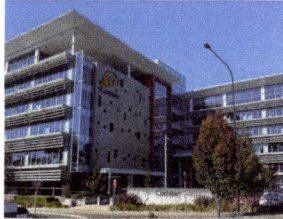

Cochlear Australia's global headquarters

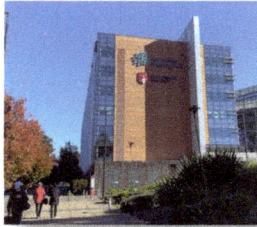

Macquarie University Hearing Hub

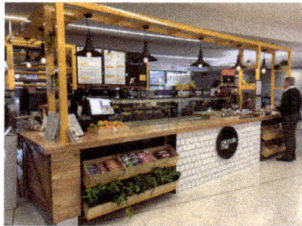

Piccolo Me MQ Hearing Hub Café

10:30 – 11:00

We entered the café and looked for our people. Our Meniere's researchers. They belonged to us. A noble type of HumanKIND filled with a passion to help others, or perhaps because they loved the academic challenge to find missing pieces to solve medical problems, maybe a mix of both. What is their story? What is their motivation? These were the bravest of brave researchers, tackling a terribly difficult disease to find solutions for, with the ultimate goal of finding a cure. They are my Meniere's Superheroes.

They stood together with an easy confidence. Smiling. Their Clark Kent personas hid their superhero status. In my curious and imaginative mind I gave them each a superhero cape. Then I joined the line to order a chai latte. I turned to see who was behind me.

'Julieann. I recognise you from our Meniere's Facebook group. I'm Mark.'

I smiled. 'Oh yeah – Mark.' And then we fell into an easy conversation. He shared his Meniere's story with me. I understood completely. He also told me how he had lost his hearing in his right ear when he was young, most probably due to the measles. A cochlear implant would change his life.

I discovered how at ease I was in the group of Menierian's. I've only met two very small groups of people with Meniere's twice in my 26 years of this awful disease. We were all the same. We had been through the same journey. We were friends, instantly. No judgement. Only sincere compassion and empathy…

The Meniere's researchers approached us and mingled while we sipped on our barista made tea, coffees, chai lattes, cappuccinos and hot chocolates, gifted to us, all paid for like we were the superheroes, and they were visiting us. I was taken back by their kindness.

11:00 – 11:30
We walked to the Lecture Theatre on Level 1. The door opened to

the impressive lecture room. I gazed up at the pitched floor with rows and rows of seats. It took me back to my own university days, and indeed of a teaching room at the school where I taught. I eased myself into the seat with a quiet confidence, keen to hear about their research.

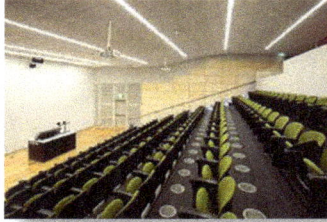

Professor David McAlpine, the director of Meniere's Disease Research at the Macquarie University Australian Hearing Hub, awardee of the prestigious Einstein Fellowship, welcomed us to the Macquarie University and reminded us of our program today. He then introduced us to the Meniere's Research Team, who are building a pipeline to cure Meniere's, bringing together a global-leading team: Dr Chris Pastras, Associate Professor Mohsen Asdina, Associate Professor Payal Mukherjee ENT (who was unable to attend), and then he added … *you*. He spoke of the importance of listening to people with Meniere's disease. They want to help *us*, and they can't do it without *our* involvement. Future tours and information sharing will continue with open invitations, as today's was.

I sat there in awe as he drew us into his world of research, our world of Meniere's, my memory cells bursting with Meniere's information, soaking in every single word, enraptured by the Professors McAlpine's passion for research and trying to cure, or at the very least, find solutions to symptoms so Meniere's people can live a quality life again.

And then came the words that had me in a spin. He told

us about an *implantable device* that will allow us to *turn off the vertigo and restore our balance.*

I couldn't stop myself from mouthing "WOW!"

I held my breath and shifted in my seat as my eyes pooled with tears. Then I inhaled deeply to calm myself.

This ... is what we have been waiting for: to be able to control our vertigo without the destruction of hearing cells, without sac decompression, without the use of gentamicin, without having a vestibular nerve section. To have an implantable device that acts like a switch to turn off the vertigo ... mind officially blown.

An answered prayer.

This is a life changer. This is a life giver.

This means finding our self again, the one before the physical, social, emotional and psychological broken pieces of us after Meniere's disease entered our lives uninvited, causing unbelievable destruction to our sense of self – who we were, our self-worth, taking our happiness, our confidence, our friends, our social lives, our enjoyment of being able to eat whatever we wanted, our ability to take part in any physical activity offered to us.

Dr Chris Pastras Dr Chris Pastras (sydney.edu.au) presented next.

Discovery:
Finding the cause of vertigo attacks in Meniere's
- Clinical Indicators
- Origin of Dysfunction
- Pathophysiology

Discovery:
A holistic pathway from discovery to translation
1. Uncover the link between endolymphatic hydrops and MD.
2. Characterise the cause of vertigo attacks for future treatments.
3. Develop novel therapeutic strategies in animal models.
4. Develop novel diagnostic tools for clinics.
5. Improve current diagnostic and treatment strategies.
6. A vestibular implant for balance rehabilitation after surgery.

Professor Mohsen Asadnia Mohsen Asadniaye Fard Jahromi — Macquarie University (mq.edu.au) followed Dr Chris Pastras.

Innovation:
Engineering novel micro/nano devices:
1. Develop devices to monitor potassium and formation of endolymph hydrops which would warn the patient of an impending MD attack, allow activation of smart drug delivery systems and help to understand the progress and severity of the disease.
2. Artificial endolymphatic sac to replenish and ionically modulate endolymph.
3. Development of highly sensitive potassium sensor.
4. Inner ear fluid – make an implantable sensor to change the ion concentrate – potassium.
5. Make an artificial sac to eliminate Meniere's – has been tested and published.
6. They have made a membrane that only lets potassium pass through.

Professor David McAlpine thanked our presenters and we applauded. His passion for everything that had been spoken about today and about Macquarie University and their cutting edge science applied to Meniere's was eagerly absorbed by me, and my imaginary bucket I brought along to fill with hope from today was already full. Wagging school for the day was totally worth the guilt of missing class with my students, but also knowing that they were in good hands with another teacher who would follow the plans I had left them.

11:30 AM-12:30 PM- Australian Hearing Hub's lab visit
We left the lecture room and followed Professor David to our next stop on the tour. It was the Australian Hearing Hub Lab. The door opened and we entered the lab room of cochlear implant innovation and ground breaking research.

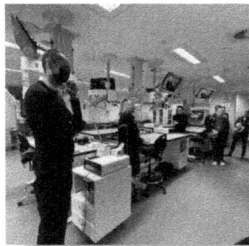

This room was named after Professor Bill Gibson who is a renowned ear, nose and throat (ENT) surgeon and world leader in cochlear implantation and Menière's disease. My heart glowed. It was Professor Bill Gibson, whom my own ENT phoned to ask for advice before he administered my gentamicin back in 2004. It was Professor Bill Gibson, who read my Meniere's novel, *The Colour of Broken* in 2018, and invited me to the Meniere's Symposium in Sydney, 2018. It was Professor Bill Gibson, whom I emailed to apologise for curing Meniere's in my new novel, *All the Colours Above* (2021), with nanorobotics, to which he replied, 'I am interested in using nanorobotics to deliver medication to the endolymphatic sac. Mohsen Asadnia is an engineer who is very interested in Meniere's disease and is a leader in nanorobotics. You can google him. He is also building models to explain the cause of the vertigo.'

Two cochlear researchers spoke. My apologies that I can't acknowledge them by name, but I was in system overload with being present in a laboratory where the technology for my own cochlear implant was created once. The cochlear implant that changed my life.

After looking around at the equipment, and the very place where cochlear implant surgeons from all around the world come to learn how to perform cochlear implant surgery, or where they watch live demonstrations on donated body parts from people who kindly give their physical body over to medical science after death, my eyes found the researchers again. More superheroes.

We saw the inner cochlear implant device that is placed under the skin on your scalp, and watched how the 22 electrodes were inserted via their ear prototype used for surgery instruction.

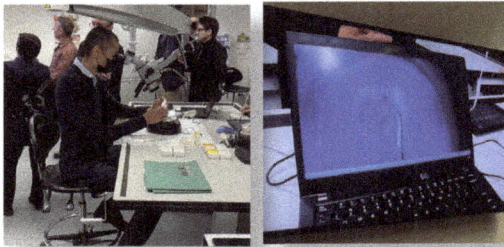

And then we were able to ask questions.

One of the people on our tour group asked about the part of the cochlear implant you wear on your head. The processor. I spoke up and showed them my Kanso 2, and how it attached to my head. After a group photo we learned about more cochlear implant research. **They are in the midst of human trials, applying hearing cell growth stimulator solution (gene therapy) into the cochlear with the electrodes at the time of the cochlear implant surgery.** The hearing cells are stimulated to grow and attach to the electrodes to improve cochlear implant hearing even further.

Watch a news snippet of the trial here: https://www.nextsense. org.au/news-and-stories/world-first-cochlear-trial-celebrates-milestone-and-calls-for-more-participants

We were also shown the half a million dollar medical robot that will be used by cochlear implant surgeons in the near future. It's an effective tool to overcome the surgeon's limitations such as tremor, drift and accurate force. They joked about how good the upcoming generation of surgeons will be at controlling the joystick of the robot with all their experience in playing video games and online gaming during their youth.

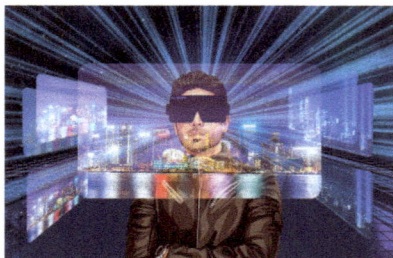

We proceeded onto the next room. On shelves were rows and rows of medical equipment and three large industrial fridges. 'Donated totally intact vestibular systems,' I was told. 'We don't want to scare you with the contents.' I wanted to tell her that's what I planned to do with my ears – to donate them to medical research to help people with Meniere's disease. I also wanted to tell her that I love biology and anatomy and the sciences, and seeing body parts like that wouldn't phase me.

We moved into a long room next. If was filled with equipment for surgeons to practise cochlear implants. Impressive. We are in good hands.

Onward bound, we entered the Anechoic Chamber – the quietest place on earth. The purpose of this room is to test sound, and to test hearing devices. The walls and ceiling was lined with fiberglass wedges. Beneath us, we stood on mesh that covered an open two floor drop below, where again the floor was covered with fibreglass wedges. This anechoic chamber at Macquarie University is the only one in the Southern Hemisphere.

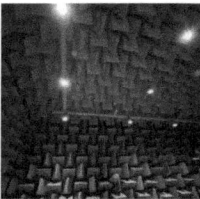

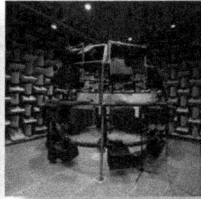

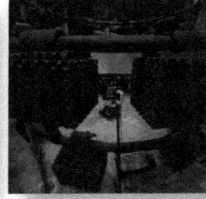

I was thrilled to be inside this space. I had read about these rooms.

Inside the room it's silent. So silent that noise is measured in negative decibels. It's a challenge for people to be in the chamber. But your ears adapt. In the absence of external sounds, you will hear your heart beating, sometimes you can hear your lungs, even hear your stomach gurgling loudly. You become the sound. If you are in the room for 30 minutes, you have to be in a chair, as people have trouble orienting themselves and even standing. It is said that the longest anybody has been able to bear it is 45 minutes.

I wondered about us Menierians. With our loud tinnitus, many with multiple unbearably loud tinnitus sounds, would we last longer than 45minutes? Those of us Menierians who have had their balance cells destroyed, would will still be able to orient ourselves and stand due to the fact that we have relearned to walk with the absence of our vestibular balance senses? I'd be open to the challenge to be in the chamber as a person with Meniere's disease. Fascinating.

12:30 PM-1 PM Lunch

I approached the long table of pre-packed lunches as a person with Meniere's disease. You know what we do, we look at the food and categorize whether it is safe for us to eat – how much salt content would be in the foods; would it give me brain fog, ear fullness, or increase the sound level of my tinnitus, would it be enough to throw me into a vertigo episode? I wondered what would be offered for lunch by the Meniere's specialists, knowing our reaction and limitations with salt. I was well pleased to find that the packaged lunch was well thought-out with our diet restrictions in mind, and so very thankful for their kindness once again. But still, when I opened the box of food, I deconstructed the Turkish bread (other types of bread were available as well) to see exactly what was on the roll (chicken, lettuce, tomato) with a side salad of carrot, celery etc, plus a chocolate roll type of bakery item. I ate what I knew wouldn't affect me.

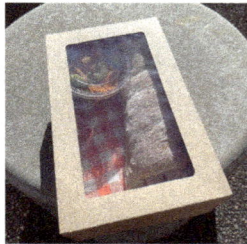

1 PM- 2 PM (Discussion and planning)

With our bellies full and Meniere's stories shared over lunch in the glorious winter sunshine (20° Celsius), we headed to another room of grouped tables and chairs for discussion and planning. This is the part of the day I was unsure about. It even made me feel a little nervous. How could we, the Meniere's sufferers, be part of planning? What could we possibly provide the highly intelligent doctors, professors and engineers, that could help them?

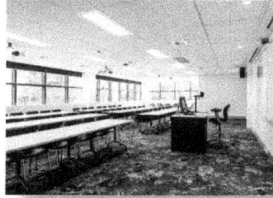

This session opened and we heard about funding for Meniere's research. Dr Romaric Bouveret – Director of Operations and Strategies spoke, as well as another guest speaker (I apologise for not recording her name). We heard that funding for Meniere's is hard to obtain, and they are actively applying for grants, once again. We also heard that Meniere's comes under the umbrella of "Hearing" at the University, and so they have access to some funds through there. The sigh of relief in the room was palpable. We were also assured that any donations sent to the Macquarie University for Meniere's would be totally committed to Meniere's research.

And then *we* were given the chance to speak. At first, some of us spoke about how they may be able to find ways to donate money – this is a hard thing to do when Meniere's has stolen your means of income.

I, too, joined this thread. I spoke about my two Meniere's novels, *The Colour of Broken* and *All the Colours Above,* that I have donated a substantial amount of money to research from sales, as well as the *Daily Meniere's Journal.*

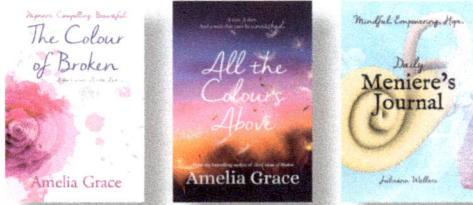

I spoke about the impact of having a story with a main character with Meniere's, and that a young girl in the US gave her mum a copy of *The Colour of Broken* … afterward, her mum came back to her begging for forgiveness, as she thought her daughter had been faking the symptoms. I also told the researchers that *The Colour of Broken* had been long listed, twice, to be made into a movie.

Awareness for us.
For Meniere's.

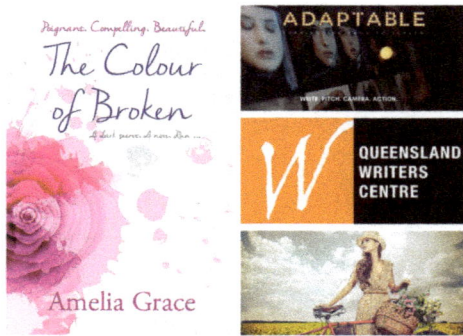

Professor David McAlpine stated the importance of the Arts (writing, art, drama, music, dance, movies, film and television) for helping to raise awareness and funds. And that collaboration across fields was important. That connection to people was important, and the Arts helps us to do that.

Then with tears, I spoke about how I've talked Meniere's

sufferers online, out of suiciding. I don't know if they wanted to hear that. But they *needed* to hear that. They need to know how Meniere's affects the lives and hearts and souls of people. They need to know how destructive it is. We want our lives back. Can you please help us?

Dr Matthieu Recugnat spoke to us next. He talked about tinnitus. He talked about hearing research, and he talked about a program they have created called *Tinnibot*, (Tinnibot Hearing Power) the world's first virtual coach (an app) that provides tinnitus support anytime, anywhere.

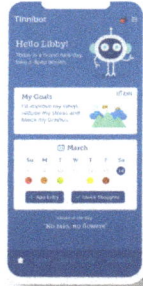

Professor Dave McAlpine asked, what else do we need?

We know that they want to hear *our* stories. Our *voice*. But we want to hear *theirs* too. What inspired them to research Meniere's disease? What drives them to do what they do? What frustrates them? What have they had successes with? Are there funny happenings at any time?

I suggested they build a website that keeps people up-to-date with the latest research. I think it's important to keep in touch with the researchers, and making connections by hearing the stories of real people, including the Meniere's research team stories.

2 PM -2:30 PM (Cochlear building visit)

Unfortunately we had gone overtime with the discussion and planning. And yet there was so much more to say. It was decided that the Cochlear building visit would have to be included in the next tour. I'll be there.

2:30 PM – End of the tour

I think I can speak for all of the Menierians present today – we are in awe of you, and so, so, so thankful.

My request for tours in the future:
To the Macquarie University -
• Record the tour sessions so they can be shared globally (with captions) – every word and every bit of added humour was precious.

As I catch my flight back to Brisbane, finally I slow down. My heart is breaking, and yet, it is full of joy. How can it be in two states at once? It's breaking because people are still suffering terribly with Meniere's disease. And yet it is full of joy. The future for us is looking bright. I know our cure, or resolutions of our symptoms is coming soon.

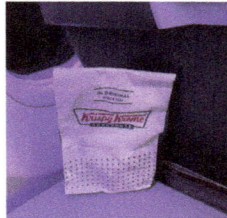

I tuck into my "traditional flight home Krispy Kremes", and reflect on the day, and hope that, while Dr David McAlpine and Dr Mohsen Asadnia are at the 2nd Inner Ear Disorders

Therapeutics Summit in Boston in two weeks to share their research and findings, and to listen to other researchers on their discoveries, all the pieces of the Meniere's jigsaw puzzle will be found.

The spark of hope can never be extinguished.

A Cochlear Implant is ...
learning to re-hear

There was only one way
to learn to hear with a cochlear implant,
and that was to use it.

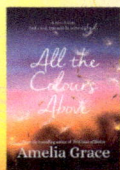

Tips for Success with a Cochlear Implant

- *Be committed.* Make time everyday to follow the exercises set by your cochlear audiologist. You are training your brain to relearn to hear.
- *Be committed to keeping all of your appointments* for mapping and updates. This is the only way to get the best possible results with your cochlear implant and to reach your full potential.
- *Ask family and friends to help* you with some listening exercises. Even if it is only 10 minutes a day.
- *Include your auditory training into activities you do each day*, for instance, while vacuuming, listen to a podcast, or while preparing food, listen to an audiobook.
- *Don't give up.* It's hard work at first, and mentally tiring. You may think you are not making any gains, but somehow, your brain slots all the pieces together like a jigsaw puzzle so your hearing will make sense.
- *Wear your cochlear implant processor everyday* for as long as

you can. I wore mine from the moment I woke up to the moment I went to bed at night.

- *Celebrate the successes*, no matter how small.
- *Practise thankfulness*, even for the littlest of things.
- *Ask for help* when you need it - from other cochlear implant users or your cochlear audiologist. If you have a problem, there is always a solution.
- *Join online cochlear implant groups.*
- *Meet up* with other cochlear implant recipients if you can.
- *Use a mini microphone.* It will help you to understand speech more clearly in background noise, like in a restaurant, decreasing your effort to listen and reducing fatigue. I also like to use the *forward focus* feature on my Nucleus Smart App.
- *Ensure you do direct streaming* to your cochlear implant to help with understanding speech and other sounds.
- *Have patience.*
- *Be kind to yourself.*
- *Take breaks* if needed.
- *Talk to yourself* about what you are doing - listening to your words to help learn speech.
- *Repetition* consolidates learnings.
- *Listen to music.*
- Do not be afraid to ask people to *repeat their words.*
- Remember that *all people have difficulty in noisy environments.* You may even find that you can hear better than them because of your cochlear implant.
- *Concentration* is very important. Pay attention.
- Concentrate on *what is said.*
- *Observe the talker*: lips, gestures, body language.
- *Plan ahead:* Think about possible challenges and plan

what to do if they occur.

- *Research* cochlear implant hearing to enhance your understanding of the process of learning to hear.
- *Listen* to other people's success stories.

Some Apps

I have listed the apps I used for learning to hear, and continue to visit to practise my cochlear implant hearing. There are many more apps to help you with your learning to hear journey than I have listed here. Your particular cochlear implant brand will also have learning to hear apps to help you.

- Join your local library so you can download audiobooks. I chose the audiobook for print books I already had at home so I could follow the printed text while listening. *Borrowbox* is what I use in Australia. Check out what your local library has in your country.
- Children's picture books are highly recommended. *Storyline Online* https://www.storylineonline.net/
- *Cochlear CoPilot*
- *Hearoes* https://www.games4hearoes.com/ FREE
- *Angelsound* http://angelsound.tigerspeech.com/ FREE
- *Hear Coach*
- *Soundscape*
- Advanced Bionics *Clix*
- *Read My Quips*
- *Word Success* App (AB)
- *Overdrive* (online ebooks and audiobooks for free)
- *Librivox* (Free public domain audiobooks)
- *The Listening Room*

Cochlear Implants and Music

Music is the most complex and sophisticated form of sound possible. The good news is that the ability to enjoy music again is within our grasp. But it does take patience and practise at listening to music. I have discovered that the cello sounds amazing with direct streaming to my CI, as well as other instruments. Here are some things I have done and apps I use to help improve my music hearing:

- I started compiling my own *Spotify* Cochlear Music Collection. I discovered, that if I already knew the song, it was easier to understand the music with direct streaming to my cochlear implant. Your music memories before hearing loss will help you.
- *Bring Back the Beat* App
- https://www.risingsoftware.com/auralia *Ear training with real music*
- Obtain the lyrics to vocal songs and follow them as you listen to the music.
- Listen repeatedly to music you were familiar with, before branching out to unknown music.
- https://cochlearimplantbasics.com/music-rehab/
- *Meludia Melody* - Ear training App
- Research other programs and Apps

The future is looking bright for hearing loss. Not only do we have cochlear implants, but these are being refined for better hearing as technology allows.

I'm also excited about the research going on for regrowth of hearing cells.

Good things are coming.

The spark of hope can never be extinguished.

My Now, 2022

My cochlear implant did change my life. **1000%**
Here's the best parts when I am wearing the processor:

- I forget that I am deaf in my left ear. It **IS** that good!
- I feel balanced in myself. A feeling of freedom.
- Listening to music with my CI ear and my good gives me a natural addictive high - I never expected that.
- I found my confidence again.
- I can hear better than other hearing people in noisy social settings at times.
- I don't have to keep asking people to repeat themselves.
- People have no idea I am hearing impaired, and treat me as a normal person.
- When I am wearing the processor, I feel safe when out and about. I don't need to have my senses on hyper alert for fear of something happening that I can't locate the sound of. That state of alertness was always draining of mentally and physically. Outings are more relaxing.
- I have direction of hearing - this is a safety feature.
- I can direct stream music or podcasts to my cochlear implant while I am working, and no one knows.
- I tell my students at school that I can hear what they think! At first they always believe me (the look on their faces is priceless). It makes them think for a moment, before I let them off the hook. Luckily they have a sense of humour.
- I have an advantage of being able to use my lip and body language reading skills as well as hearing speech. This is a insight into others, and a gift of seeing the truth.

In my future ...

For my cochlear implant ear:
- I will continue updating the technology as it comes out.
- I will continue to go to mappings as my audiologist requests, and if I think I need my cyborg hearing to be checked.
- I will continue to revisit hearing exercises, even when I think I am doing well.

For my "good" ear that has hearing loss:
- I am following hearing cell regrowth research, and when it is ready, I will be putting my hand up for the procedure, just like Scarlett in my novel, *All the Colours Above*. If it doesn't eventuate, I will not hesitate in getting another cochlear implant.

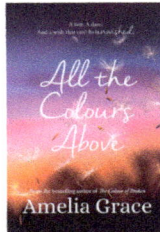

I write this book with the knowledge of the great diversity of experiences of people with Meniere's disease, cochlear implants and acknowledging that there are many debilitating incurable illnesses, and I am in not in any way discrediting or minimalising another person's illness.

I'm looking forward to the day when I hear: 'Here's the bad news. You have Meniere's disease. Here's the good news—we can fix it!'

I'm looking forward to the day when I hear: 'Here's the bad news. You have hearing loss. Here's the good news—we can fix it!'

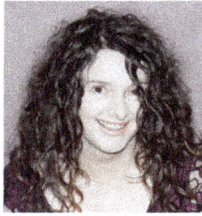

Julieann Wallace is a multi-published author and artist. When she is not disappearing into her imaginary worlds as *Julieann Wallace* – children's author, or as *Amelia Grace* – fiction novelist, she is working as a Secondary Arts Teacher. Julieann's 7th novel with a main character with Meniere's disease—*The Colour of Broken*—written under her pen name of Amelia Grace, was #1 on Amazon in its category a number of times, and was longlisted to be made into a movie or TV series by *Screen Queensland, Australia*, twice. Her 8th novel has a Deaf character, who has a cochlear implant and is trialling hearing cell regrowth.

Julieann donates profits from her books to Macquarie University, where they are researching Meniere's disease to find a cure. Julieann is a self-confessed tea ninja and Cadbury chocoholic, has a passion for music and art, and tries not to scare her cat, Claude Monet, with her terrible cello playing.

https://www.julieannwallaceauthor.com/
https://www.facebook.com/julieannwallace.author
https://www.instagram.com/julieann_wallace_/
https://www.instagram.com/myshadow_menieres/

Acknowledgements

Thank you to my friend, *Dave Mujunen*, who encouraged me to make the step to get a cochlear implant, telling me it would "change my life!" It did. Thank you for your wise words.

An enormous thank you to *Vivek*. You inspired me to get my own cochlear implant.

A BIG thank you, again, to *my husband*, for his forever support and understanding that writing is the only place where I can escape from my Meniere's disease - 27 years at the time of printing this novel, since that day changed my life for my earth time. (Dx:1995)

My three beautiful children, thank you for all you do. And thank you for holding my hand during the torturous violent vertigo where I would stare at the wall for hours and hours at a time, and as adults, thank you for listening to me rant on about my writing or wacky ideas that pop into my head, and for your compassion as you watched my tears fall as I struggled with life, or was overcome with emotion from readers thanking me for writing *The Colour of Broken*. I am indeed blessed.

A heartfelt thank you to my dear *mum and dad*, who always dropped everything the moment I went into a violent spinning session for at least 4 hours at a time (I used to call it a SPAT – spinning attack), which was often, and they would come to take care of my three kids while I was totally debilitated. I will eternally cherish your love and support. And thank you for your support for me as I went through my cochlear implant journey.

Thank you to my team of *medical doctors*, Dr. Ann Masjakin (GP), Dr. Maurice Stevens (ENT), Dr. Christopher Que Hee (ENT and CI Surgeon), Professor Graeme Clark, who pioneered the Multi-channel Cochlear Implant, my Cochlear Audiologist,

Karen Pedley, who fine-tunes my cochlear hearing at "mapping" sessions by connecting me to a computer, and to the legendary, Emeritus Prof Bill Gibson AO aka The Meniere's Guru ... 'Look for the helpers!' - you are the helpers! Thank you for your extraordinary care.

And to you, *the reader* of this book, and to *my friends* and *family*, thank you for choosing to read my cochlear implant story. It means more to me than you can ever know!

Finally, thank you to my *Creator*, for always carrying me through the terrifying storm, for giving me hope when it felt like there was none, and for giving me a Light to hold onto in the darkness so I could find my way back home.

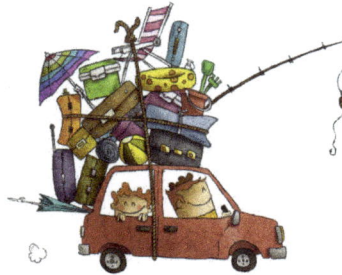

.